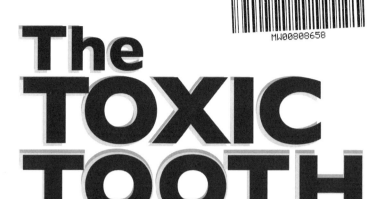

The TOXIC TOOTH

How a root canal could be making you sick

Robert Kulacz, DDS and
Thomas E. Levy, MD, JD

with a Foreword by:
Boyd E. Haley, PhD

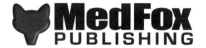

MedFox
PUBLISHING

Dedicated to
George E. Meinig, DDS, FACD (1914-2008),
a tireless patient advocate and author of
Root Canal Cover-Up

ACKNOWLEDGMENTS

As I have in the past, I want to thank my wife, Lis, and my daughter, Daniela, for making me so important in their lives and allowing me to live my life to the fullest. I especially want to thank my dear Mother, who passed away just before this book was published, as she has always been my number one friend, and she has always given me the most support for all my endeavors in life. I never did anything that I did not discuss with her first. Also, my sister, Cathy, has always been a strong source of comfort and support for me as well.

My good friend and colleague, Ron Hunninghake, has continued his invaluable support in allowing me to discuss and properly analyze any wild thought that comes into my head. So many of my thoughts would never have evolved without him.

Thomas E. Levy, MD, JD

The love and support of my wife Susan continues to give me the strength to never waver in my search for the truth. You got more than you bargained for when you married me; thank you for believing in me. My daughters Jackie and Jenna who let me be a kid again. You always make me proud.

To Bob Bull who has dramatically improved my tennis game: Thanks for being a great friend. Pretty soon I will beat you in a match!

And to all my other friends at Saw Mill Club, Steve and Lynne Levine, Lori Stern, Joe Bottino, Paul Cantor, Kevin Kane, Donna

Arena, Miles Slater, Tom Formichella, Peter DeJong, for your encouragement and humor. I am very lucky to have you all in my life. To Marc and Nancy Epstein, you understand me and still like me, so thanks!

Robert Kulacz, DDS

———————— *Mutual Acknowledgments* ————————

Thanks and a great deal of gratitude are extended to Les and Cindy Nachman, without whom this book would not be a reality. And finally, a big thanks to Dave Nicol, who could not be a better editor. We often ended up expanding upon his thoughts, rather than just having him package our thoughts better. The book is enormously better because of him.

TABLE of CONTENTS

CHAPTER EIGHT
Before My Own Eyes   201
• EXPERIENCES *with Root Canal Treatment*

CHAPTER NINE
Some Healthy Options   231
• ALTERNATIVES *to Root Canal Treatment*

This book by Drs. Kulacz and Levy should be required reading for all physicians and dentists. First, all the research that I have read over the years has supported the ideas of Dr. Weston Price that doing root canals on teeth makes them susceptible to multiple types of infection by bacteria that cause different systemic type infections. Dr. Price's research was brilliant for its time.

However, the discoveries of Dr. Price caused problems for an area of dentistry called endodontics that was developing into a very lucrative business. His research was actively attacked by those who wanted no discussion on the safety of their money-making procedures. However, a Dr. George Meinig, one of the early endodontists who had issues with the root canal procedure's safety, wrote a book called "Root Canal Cover-Up" which brought more to the forefront of the health dangers of the root canal procedure with regards to the causation link to multiple systemic infections.

Both Dr. Price and Dr. Meinig were attacked by their peers who wanted to maintain the illusion of root canals being safe. Dr. Kulacz is just one of the latest to feel the unjustified wrath of the Endodontic profession for asserting that infected, root canal-treated teeth could be the focal source for remote infections. Such infections, caused by the delivery of microbes from the infected teeth into the bloodstream, end up in specific organs and sites throughout the body, resulting in various systemic illnesses.

I was personally introduced to this issue through my involvement in the likely toxicological problems caused by mercury vapor escaping from dental amalgams. Dr. Hal Huggins informed me that the toxicity from teeth with root canals was much worse than the mercury vapor from an amalgam-filled tooth. I didn't at all believe him but he insisted that I check out some teeth that he had extracted from patients, some with and some without root canals.

My research assistants were startled at the level of toxicity against brain enzymes that was observed by merely placing the teeth into distilled water and then testing the ability of this "tooth treated water" to inhibit or kill important enzymes found in brain tissue. From this initial simple testing we developed a procedure to test both teeth and gum-related crevicular fluid for toxic effects. The overall finding can be summarized by stating that dead tissue like root canal-treated teeth, if left in the body, will become infected with pathogenic bacteria, and this infection can, and usually does, spread to other parts of the body. When we tested teeth with root canals sent to us by dentists we never found a tooth that wasn't toxic to some degree. However, some were extremely toxic indicating that they were capable of sending bacteria and exotoxins to other body locations that could cause extreme illnesses.

We were challenged by endodontists that this translocation of infective microbes could not and did not occur since some endodontists had attempted to prove Dr. Price's "focal infection theory" to be invalid years earlier. In my opinion, the science that "proved" Dr. Price wrong was very questionable and poorly done. However, a recent technology that won its inventor a Nobel Prize in Science, called Polymerase Chain Reaction or PCR, came into play and has provided incredible scientific support to Dr. Price's focal infection theory. Simply stated, PCR can identify the infectious bacteria found to cause multiple systemic infections such as placenta infections leading to preterm labor and low birth weight, infections in atherosclerotic plaques leading to heart attacks, as well as multiple infections found in various organs like the kidneys, liver, etc.

This is not an outrageous concept, as bacteria from the oral cavity are basically the primary source of bacteria causing most systemic infections. The presence of dead, root canal-treated teeth, with the high levels of pathogenic bacteria formed within them from the oral cavity, greatly enhances the delivery of pathogenic microbes and exotoxins into the body. PCR studies have many times identified the source of pathogenic bacteria found in infected organs as being the same as found in root canal-treated teeth from the same patient. To deny this is absurd posturing—but it is done by those who wish to continue making a living by inflicting their patients with dangerous root canals.

Teeth with root canals also lead to jawbone osteonecrosis or cavitations that harbor the same pathogenic microbes that start out in the dead tooth. Cavitations can cause immense pain and suffering as well as donate microbial infections to cause systemic illnesses. In the time that I tested teeth and debris from cavitations for toxicity I found many teeth with root canals that had lower toxin levels than seen in cavitations. However, I never found any cavitation-derived material that was not extremely toxic to the test enzymes we used.

Over time, I became known to many patients that were treated for this toxicity by removal of teeth with root canals and extraction of the cavitational debris by oral surgery. Considering that this was the initial phase of many dentists trying to help their patients survive the systemic illnesses caused by questionable dental procedures, the success rate was quite impressive. The very scientific PCR studies show that they were on the right track. Yet even today there is strong denial from the Endodontic societies that root canals can lead to systemic infections and disease, and much of the strong scientific proof of the root canal-induced toxicity is ignored. Those that would reveal it are doing so at great personal risk for their professional lives. This book by Drs. Kulacz and Levy details this current struggle.

Dr. Boyd Haley
Professor Emeritus
Department of Chemistry
University of Kentucky,
Lexington, KY

Boyd E. Haley, PhD
CTI Science

The High Price of Rocking the Boat

Robert Kulacz, DDS

When the New York State Office of Professional Discipline (OPD) began investigating my dental practice in 2005, I realized that there were many dentists who disagreed with me. I had once been where they were, completely immersed in a busy dental practice and totally unaware of the comprehensive and compelling research that exposes the systemic risks of root canal treatments.

At first, I allayed my nagging fears with a naive confidence. Surely these investigators were guided by a sincere concern for the public in general and my patients specifically. Once all the science, the microbiological cultures, the pathology reports, the X-rays, and the nearly miraculous patient outcomes were clearly set before them, their eyes, previously blinded by ignorance, would be opened—even as mine had been many years before. Ultimately the OPD would vindicate me and even embrace my practice of dentistry.

Boy, was I wrong!

I was soon to discover that these investigators, who were supposedly truth-seeking advocates for patient welfare, were no more interested in uncovering the truth than a cop who's paid to look the other way.

When the decision was made to write this new book, I was not planning to recount the incredibly painful history that started with the OPD's initial contact. However, friends encouraged me. They felt it would provide a reality check glimpse into the consequence of challenging long-accepted clinical paradigms of the American Dental Association. Plus, and maybe even more importantly, it could help explain the resistance patients will get from their general dentist or endodontist when they question the safety of root canal-treated teeth.

My journey began when a patient told me that his doctor had warned him against root canal therapy.

Before the realities presented in this book invaded my world, I performed dentistry just like the majority of dentists do. Life was good. I enjoyed what I did and I made a decent living from it. I was exactly where I wanted to be in life. I worked 4.5 days per week and made enough money to do just about anything that I wanted to do. I took flying lessons and got my pilot's license. I bought a house. I bought an aerobatic airplane and flew it three or four times a week. I had a wonderful family and my wife and I were thoroughly enjoying raising our twin girls.

Life was great. I had arrived.

I often ask myself why I rocked the boat when everything was going so well. Frankly, I do not have an answer that provides me much comfort. I suppose I just felt obligated to go in whatever direction the scientific truth led me. At the same time I certainly understand much better the reasons why many other dentists would never even consider such a path.

My journey began when a patient told me that his doctor had warned him against root canal therapy, and that this procedure could initiate a wide range of medical diseases.

I quickly retorted, "That's ridiculous, whoever said that is completely crazy. You shouldn't listen to such nonsense!"

It made me angry that someone in the medical field would propagate this absurdity. I felt personally attacked so I began to research the validity of these claims in order to prove to my patient that his physician was wrong.

My quest led me to the works of Weston Price, Edward Rosenow, and Frank Billings, all pioneers in the early research clearly linking dental infections to systemic disease. Although I found their research very interesting, I just "knew" that these writings from the 1920's were "ancient" and had certainly been disproved with more contemporary research.

Then I went to an International Academy of Oral Medicine and Toxicology meeting where I attended a lecture by Professor Boyd Haley. At that time Dr. Haley was the department chair of chemistry at The University of Kentucky. He spoke about the toxicity that he found in *all* root canal-treated teeth and the detrimental inhibition of key bodily enzymes that had been demonstrated by testing the toxins released from these teeth. I felt like I had been punched in the stomach. Could this be true?

I searched in vain for any scientific studies that refuted the research of Price, Rosenow, Billings, and the evidence presented by Haley. To be fair, there were a few editorial articles in the *Journal of the American Dental Association* that were critical of these earlier scientists. However, rather than provide research or data to substantiate the position of the American Dental Association (ADA), these editorials attempted to discredit previous researchers on their experimental techniques. These articles never addressed the huge volume of data that had been independently amassed by these diligent scientists; they completely sidestepped the research demonstrating the risks of the root canal procedure.

What a blow to my professional pride. I didn't like what I had discovered, but I couldn't deny the powerful evidence. My patient was right and I was wrong.

Contrary to what I had been taught, I was forced to conclude that root canal treatment was not a benign procedure without systemic health risks. In good conscience, I could no longer practice dentistry as I had learned it. I had to change the focus of my practice.

I knew that I if I were to best treat patients who were coming to see me, I had to learn a lot more about the intersection of dentistry and medicine. To satisfy this need for knowledge, I read through countless journal articles and consulted a number of medical textbooks.

Many of my patients noticed great improvement in medical conditions that had been plaguing them for years.

During that time, many of the patients that I saw had migrated through a series of doctors without resolution of their medical conditions. Although I was in no way qualified to treat their wide variety of ailments, I wanted to know as much as I could about all aspects of medicine. I was convinced that the disconnect between dentistry and medicine was arbitrary, and was potentially harmful to patients. These disciplines needed to be integrated, and I wanted to work hand-in-hand with my patients' physicians, knowing that my work could help improve their overall health.

It was not long before all of my time was devoted to treating acute and chronic oral infections. Many of my patients noticed great improvement in medical conditions that had been plaguing them for years, and my practice grew simply by word of mouth.

I did not treat everyone who came to see me. In fact, I turned away the majority of those who wanted surgery because they simply did not need it or they had unrealistic expectations about the outcome.

It would soon become clear that scientific validity and positive patient outcomes were irrelevant to them.

Never did I treat patients' medical conditions or even suggest that their medical conditions were caused by a root canal-treated tooth or cavitation. I simply told them that I would surgically remove the dead and infected bone. If the tissue biopsies and microbiology cultures indicated that they needed additional antibiotic therapy, I would continue to treat them, but usually only after consulting with their physicians.

At times patients needed no further treatment. At other times the tissue biopsy and microbiological cultures revealed infection and inflammation with some highly pathogenic, antibiotic-resistant microorganisms. Some of these were resolved with an oral course of an antibiotic while a few others required longer term, intravenous antibiotic therapy.

While my extraction fees were higher than those of most dentists, my pre-op consultation and extraction procedure was far more extensive. Often treatment included surgical tooth removal, biopsy and culture of all surgical sites, removal of the dead or diseased tissue in the bone around the residual tooth socket (debridement), and placement of antibiotic-impregnated graft material. These procedures were far more involved and time-consuming than traditional extractions. So even though I charged more for the treatment, my net income was about half what I made when I was practicing all phases of dentistry. Contrary to the claims of some of my critics, it was **never** about the money.

As my oral infection treatment protocol became well known, I began to do a weekly radio show on Healthy Talk Radio with host Deborah Ray. I enjoyed speaking about various dental topics, and I was astounded by the wide range of dental experiences of the listeners who called into the show. It was at that time that I decided to write a book on the systemic effects of oral infections, mainly because I wanted a reference for my patients who wanted to learn more about this subject.

I asked Dr. Tom Levy if he would be interested in writing the book with me. I had met him a few years earlier and was very impressed by his knowledge and understanding of this topic. Thankfully, he said yes and *The Roots of Disease* was completed and published in 2002.

The popularity of the radio show and the book greatly expanded my public exposure and made me a prime target for attack by the dental boards. Any individual who speaks up and questions the belief system of an organization should expect that organization to retaliate. And although I had known of other dentists who were targeted by the dental board for practicing similarly, I naively felt secure. After all, I had a very detailed informed consent form, and I never talked anyone into a procedure. In fact, I talked more people out of treatment than I actually treated. I had pathology reports and microbiological cultures confirming infection in all the teeth and surrounding bone that I removed, and I had the science to back up all of my treatment decisions.

However, as admitted to me by the OPD attorney, none of this was of interest to the dental board. It would soon become clear that scientific validity and positive patient outcomes were irrelevant to them. They had a completely different agenda.

The New York State Dental Board began an investigation regarding the extraction of two root canal-treated teeth in one of my former patients. They requested a copy of my patient's chart and all X-rays. I was a little concerned but I knew that my treatment was correct, and I felt confident that after review of the data it would be very clear that there was no basis for any disciplinary action.

A short time later, to my surprise, I received a letter from the OPD charging me with two counts of gross misconduct. The first was for the "negligent extraction" of two root canal-treated teeth, and the other accused me of an ethics violation. The dental board claimed that the statement on my website: "I changed the focus of my practice after learning of some of the dangers in dental procedures," implied a claim of superiority over other dentists. By their interpretation, this was a direct violation of the code of ethics.

The penalty for these violations:
Revocation of my license!

They were determined to revoke my license for extracting two infected root canal-treated teeth. One tooth had previously undergone an apicoectomy, which is a procedure done after an earlier root canal treatment has failed. The other tooth had a vertical fracture. Pathology from both these surgical sites *confirmed infection* of both teeth as well as chronic osteomyelitis of the surrounding bone. Microbiological cultures showed multiple species of bacteria from the infected jawbone. The facts of the case were so clear-cut that even a non-dentist could have seen that my treatment was 100% appropriate and in the best health interests of the patient.

It is interesting to note that a patient can choose to have either a root canal procedure or an extraction when seeing a dentist for an infected tooth. If the patient chooses to have an extraction instead of a root canal procedure there is absolutely no professional misconduct. However, a patient cannot change his or her mind after the root canal procedure is completed. Any dentist who extracts the treated tooth can be brought up on charges of misconduct.

This is absurd. It would be misconduct if a dentist talked a person into having a root canal-treated tooth extracted that the patient wanted to keep. However, that was absolutely not the case in my situation. The patient specifically sought me out for the sole purpose of having me extract two root canal-treated teeth that showed X-ray evidence of pathology. The patient even sent me letters after the extractions praising me for what I was doing.

Immediately, I consulted my malpractice insurance carrier to obtain coverage for my legal defense, and they stated that these charges were not covered by my policy. I was on my own.

Even so, I was still confident that once I presented all the data to the OPD, the charges would be dropped. Yes, I had spoken out against one of the most lucrative procedures in dentistry, and it was not hard to imagine why the dental board was motivated to discredit me and remove me from practice. But I still had hope that the attorneys at the OPD would be able to objectively see that I had done nothing wrong.

I contacted the OPD prosecuting attorney assigned to my case, and we began discussions about how the OPD would proceed. I sent him numerous scientific references supporting my treatment approaches. Many of my patients wrote letters on my behalf to the dental board.

After review, he said that the board had not reversed its initial decision and that the OPD was intent on full prosecution. I was sickened and disheartened as I began to realize the hopelessness of my predicament.

Some time later he called and asked me to schedule an informal settlement conference. This was to be a simple meeting where the defendant meets with the OPD representatives to discuss the penalty. He asked me what my available days were to schedule this. I told him that the only time that I could not make this meeting was on Tuesday mornings.

A short time later he called me and told me that the informal settlement conference was scheduled for a Tuesday morning. I reminded him that Tuesday was the only time that I told him I could not attend. Several days later I called him back and told him that I rearranged my schedule and that I could now attend that Tuesday morning meeting.

That was no longer an option. He told me that my slot was "taken." I asked to be rescheduled for the next available time but he told me that this would "not be possible." He said that since I initially stated that I was not able to attend the assigned conference my slot was given away and that no other appointments would be assigned. It had already been decided: the revocation of my license would be the penalty.

There was never even a pretense of fair play in this process. It was clear that their singular plan was to strip me of my license. And since a license to practice a profession is considered a privilege and not a right—even though obtaining such a license involves a lifetime of hard work and sacrifice—there are no guarantees of due process, a fair trial, or "innocent until proven guilty." The Dental Board and the OPD are not bound by the same rules as the American legal system.

I wanted to know exactly who was behind this attack on me so I filed a Freedom of Information Act (FOIA) request about my case to see exactly how the case against me was put together and who was making these decisions that would have such a profound impact on my life.

The request was denied. Apparently, the New York State Board of Regents has exempted itself from the Freedom of Information Act and does not have to release anything. They can operate in complete secrecy and for whatever reasons they deem appropriate.

At that point I decided to contact my U.S. Senator, Hillary Clinton. I called her office and explained my whole story to a staff member. I sent the same documentation to her office that I sent to the dental board. Senator Clinton felt that the charges against me warranted further discussion so she wrote a letter to the OPD asking for another review of my case. Unfortunately, her letter did not even slow down the prosecution.

Shortly after, the OPD attorney called and told me that my case was going to be reviewed by three separate dentists across New York State. I requested permission to speak to these dentists. Once again, my request was denied.

Several weeks later the attorney called again. He told me that the three new dentists who reviewed my case all came to the same conclusion—that these two teeth should not have been extracted, a truly absurd conclusion based upon the pathology and microbiology reports from the surgical sites.

So I asked him, "Where are these three dentists located?" He told me that one was in New York City, one was in Long Island, and one was in the northwest region of the state.

"Alright then, if these dentists are so far apart how were they able to so quickly review the X-rays and all the data that I sent you?" I asked.

"They didn't," he responded.

"What? They didn't? They didn't even review the X-rays and they came to the same conclusion as the dental board? Who is the one really guilty of misconduct here? Is this justice?"

He knew that he had just said something that he should not have revealed to me. "Look, you're a smart guy," he said. "Forget about the truth. Forget about justice. This has nothing to do with justice. It has nothing to do with this patient. They have an agenda."

> *"Forget about justice. This has nothing to do with justice... They have an agenda."*

Suddenly, the true motives of the OPD were clear: they just wanted to silence me for good. I never had a chance.

What the attorney did not know was that I had tape-recorded many of my phone conversations with him. I was not about to let his shocking disclosure go unchallenged. I called the Chancellor for the New York State Board of Regents. I got voice mail when I called and described my situation. I proceeded to state that the State Dental Board and the OPD were both corrupt, and reiterated what the OPD attorney told me about the board's agenda. I said that I had this on tape and proceeded to play a portion of a previously recorded conversation with the OPD attorney as proof that I did record my conversations with him.

I could not afford to go back into practice, and I could not afford to pursue my legal "rights."

The next day I received a call from the attorney. He said that the board wanted to drop all charges against me if I would simply plead "guilty" to a records violation. A records violation was only a slap on the wrist but it would still allow them to protect themselves from future legal action for filing malicious prosecution.

I didn't want to accept this plea bargain, but after speaking with an attorney who handles many board actions, he advised me to take it. He said that if I had that actual recording we could pursue it. But since I did not, it would take five years and a quarter of a million dollars in legal fees; I would win, but they would find some other way to get me. So I reluctantly took the plea. In July 2006 I signed the plea agreement.

At the time it seemed like a fairly innocuous settlement. But because of this "minor" records violation, insurers immediately labeled me as "high risk" and I was denied malpractice coverage. To obtain malpractice insurance I had to go to the New York State high-risk pool. My malpractice premium, which was originally about $8,000 per year and typical for a practice performing predominately oral surgery, jumped to nearly $80,000 per year.

The OPD and its attorney had out-maneuvered me. I could not afford to go back into practice, and I could not afford to pursue my legal "rights."

The stress of this year-long process nearly killed me, and having my career ripped away so easily and so unjustly was enough to drive me crazy as well. I knew that if I went back to practice the dental board would eventually come after me again. Their victory was devastating. The idea of going through this process a second time was unthinkable. I was through with dentistry. All the years of education and building a practice and suddenly it was over. I cannot describe in words the visceral feelings that I experienced confronting this reality. I could not sleep. I could not eat. I felt so alone. What would I do? I would have to change careers. Even if I still wanted to practice dentistry, a massive malpractice premium had put that possibility out of reach.

So, as difficult as it was to accept, I decided to explore other career options. But that possibility was quickly swept off the table as well.

Because of my position on root canal treatment, the QuackWatch website wrote an article about me and posted it on the Internet. QuackWatch is a site that claims to expose fraudulent medical practices and beliefs. Some of the things that they do are good. However, in my opinion, some of its actions are simply designed to silence anyone who speaks out against mainstream medical or dental ideology.

What's more, a link to this article was on page one of Google when anyone would do a search of my name. That, along with the OPD records violation, was the first thing that people saw when they Googled my name. The impact on my reputation and my future was devastating.

I tried to apply for other jobs but never made it to the interview phase. Once, when a prospective employer Googled my name and saw the QuackWatch article and the OPD action, I was immediately rejected.

How would I ever get a job?

An attorney friend of mine said, "Why don't you change your name? Just change your name."

That idea sounded crazy at first but after thinking about it, it started to make more sense. So in 2008 I changed my name to Cole Sommers in the hope of starting fresh.

Shortly after I changed my name, QuackWatch found out and posted it on their website. The link to the article again appeared as the first listing on page one of a Google search for "Cole Sommers." The OPD also tied my new name with my records violation on their website. Now all searchers were immediately exposed to this maligning information when searching my new name on Google. The article about me on QuackWatch has finally been removed, but the OPD listing still appears on page one of a search on my name.

> *I am persuaded that an honest review of the scientific research vindicates my position.*

Even though this incredible injustice has made me angry and bitter, I harbor no ill will against my fellow dentists. I wish them no harm. But I am convinced that the health of millions is in the balance, and I am persuaded that an honest review of the scientific research vindicates my position. If the truth inconveniences dentists and changes the way dentistry is practiced around the world, then so be it. But the health and welfare of patients have to be the primary concerns.

I also understand that agencies and associations that protect the dental/endodontic industry will throw unmitigated and unrelenting force against any suggestion that root canal treatment can cause or contribute to systemic disease. Hundreds of billions of dollars are at stake—and not just for dentists, but also for the agencies/associations that represent them. If the truth about root canal treatment reaches the masses, the insurance industry could be hit with a financial tsunami as well.

"Look, you are going after the wrong guy. I feel 100% better than I did before."

How could the truth about root canal treatment impact the insurance industry? There are many potential battles. One of these will be over the definition of medical care/coverage and dental care/coverage. A recent experience reveals how this might play out...

About one year after the State Dental Board action against me was over, I received a telephone call from the New Jersey attorney general's office. An insurance company had filed a complaint against me stating that I was committing insurance fraud. They wanted to come and interview me about a former dental patient whom I had treated and for whom I had submitted a medical insurance claim. They told me the patient's name and we scheduled a time to meet.

I called the patient to ask if he knew anything about this and he told me that two investigators from the New Jersey attorney general's office had come to see him at work and asked a lot of questions about the treatment that I had performed. After a lengthy discussion with the investigators my former patient told them, "Look, you are going after the wrong guy. I feel 100% better than I did before and all my blood work is much better. Why are you going after him?"

Since I no longer had an office, the two investigators came to my home. They sat down, turned on their tape recorder, and we proceeded to review the patient's chart. We discussed my treatment, which consisted of the extraction of five upper teeth. Each of these teeth had severe infections that extended to the surrounding jawbone and into the floor of the maxillary sinus. Pathology reports showed disease present in the maxillary sinus that had originated in the jawbone surrounding these five teeth.

My treatment included removal of the five teeth, debridement of the infected jawbone, removal of the infected tissue from the sinus, and closure of the opening between the maxillary sinus and the mouth. It was an extensive surgery.

The investigator kept asking questions about the surgical procedure, especially the extraction of the teeth, stating that the extraction of teeth is strictly a dental procedure.

I told him that the extraction of the teeth was the least of this procedure. The most important part was the removal of the infected bone, the removal of the infected tissue within the sinus, and the closure of the opening between the sinus and the mouth. He kept pressing that this was dental and not medical stating that my medical code of operating on the maxillary jawbone was not valid and insisted that

this was strictly a dental and not a medical procedure.

Finally, I pulled out the panoramic X-ray and put
it on the view box. I pointed out all of the infection
within the jawbone and how it extended up into the
maxillary sinus. Then I gave him a pencil and asked
him to draw a line on the X-ray where dentistry
stopped and medicine began.

Of course he couldn't do it. A week or two later
I received a call from the investigator telling me
that the case was closed and there was no fraud or
misconduct. I was relieved and felt somewhat vindi-
cated from the ruling (see Appendix G).

As if the dental board action and the New Jersey
Attorney General's investigation were not enough,
there were also two lawyers, one in New York and
one in California, who placed ads on Craigslist and
other Internet sites soliciting patients to sue me.
One of them also contacted the hospital where I had
surgical privileges in an attempt to have these privileges revoked.

I was even included in a malpractice suit filed
against another dentist just because I had previously treated the same patient. But when the person
who filed this lawsuit against the other dentist was
deposed, she did not even know that I was included
in the lawsuit! She went on to say that she was very
happy with my treatment and could not understand
why I was being sued. This lawyer apparently had
included me in his lawsuit without her knowledge.

Concluding Thoughts

As soon as the link between root canal-treated teeth and medical conditions is appropriately accepted by mainstream medicine, surgical extractions of these teeth, along with expensive restorations, will have to be covered by health insurance, regardless of where dentistry stands on the issue. There could be class action lawsuits akin to those that were launched against the tobacco industry. And malpractice lawsuits against dentists could abound.

There could be class action lawsuits akin to those that were launched against the tobacco industry.

Who really cares if the evidence is overwhelming? Does the truth really matter? Maybe I should just shut up and sit down. Part of me wishes I could... but I just can't.

People often ask me if I would ever go back to practice. My answer is that even if the cost of malpractice insurance was affordable, I could never go back. I also ask them to read the information contained in this book, observe what has already happened to me as a result of the first book, and then ask themselves what they would do if they were me. The board action against me shattered my faith in the belief that truth always prevails. I have never been under so much stress in my life. It not only negatively affected me personally but it had a severe negative impact on my family. I simply cannot go through that again.

History is full of people who have had their lives trampled and even crushed for trying to speak the truth. Yes, I would like to clear my name. My reputation is very important to me. But, considering the money, forums, and other resources that can be employed against me, there is little hope for that during my lifetime. However, I am confident that truth will eventually prevail and provide complete vindication.

In the meantime, Tom Levy and I hope that we can help motivated readers make informed decisions about their teeth and health by presenting the growing science that confirms the risks of root canal-treated teeth. And if in the process, this "sortie" produces another crack in the false foundations upon which some aspects of modern dentistry rest, that would be welcome.

Why We Are Questioning the Safety of Root Canal Treatments—Again

> *"All truth passes through three stages. First, it is ridiculed. Second, it is violently opposed. Third, it is accepted as being self-evident."*
>
> Arthur Schopenhauer,
>
> German philosopher (1788 – 1860)

"The 'root canals cause disease' myth was debunked over 60 years ago!" So say those who vehemently defend the safety of the root canal procedure. Advocates of the root canal procedure would claim science and millions of "successful" procedures are on their side. Since the publication of *The Roots of Disease* in 2002, the dental profession has likened the authors to those in the early 20th century who believed the earth was flat.

We would like to suggest a different historical parallel...

A Frightening Lesson from a "Crazy" Doctor

In the mid-19th century, the risk of death for women having a baby delivered by a doctor in the hospital was up to 20 times higher than having it at home. Dr. Ignac Semmelweis, a Hungarian obstetrician, became distraught by the reality that he and his medical colleagues were losing nearly a third of their obstetric patients to childbed fever, which is a bacterial infection now identified as Group A hemolytic streptococcus.

Within 24 hours of giving birth, Dr. Semmelweis would often find himself in a battle to save new mothers suffering with raging fevers, vomiting, diarrhea, writhing pain, and thick pus oozing from their birth canals. Without a remedy, and virtually without exception, he helplessly watched these horrifying symptoms ravage his postpartum patients until they died. Often, other frightened, tearful patients in his obstetrics ward begged to be allowed to leave the hospital because they believed that the doctors' involvement in the birth process was somehow responsible for childbed fever and the death that almost always ensued.

Semmelweis desperately sought for answers. Over time he noticed that the doctors and students—in the teaching hospitals where this disease was alarmingly prevalent—began their workday in the hospital morgue performing autopsies on the women who had perished from childbed fever the day before.

Without washing their hands after the autopsy procedure, the doctors would begin to attend to the women in labor.

He postulated the existence of a "morbid poison" that these doctors might be passing from dead patients to those in the delivery room. Because of this observation, he insisted that all his students wash their hands before touching their patients. Immediately, the incidence of childbed fever among the patients under his care dropped precipitously. Believing that he had rightly diagnosed the source of the disease and discovered effective preventative measures, he strongly recommended hand-washing to all of his colleagues.

Without washing their hands after the autopsy procedure, the doctors would begin to attend to the women in labor.

They quickly rejected these hygienic recommendations and were highly critical of him. After all, acceptance of his theory would be an unthinkable admission that they were responsible for the deaths of thousands of women. Semmelweis' hand-washing protocol was so vehemently opposed that the rejection by his peers literally drove him crazy. He died in an asylum in 1865.

Semmelweis' concept of a "morbid poison" may seem "unscientific" compared to a more enlightened 21st century understanding of bacterial infection. But his ignorance of current day microbiology did not invalidate his call to change a universally-accepted medical practice. He rightly directed attention to a legitimate health problem. Thousands of untreated new mothers perished needlessly while his protocol was mercilessly ridiculed and virtually unheeded.

Thankfully, a century and a half later, hospital hand-washing procedures are even more stringent than Semmelweis could have ever imagined. Unfortunately, the poor doctor was never able to experience his own vindication.

Several Common Arguments Fail the Logic Test

Some would attempt to validate the safety of root canal procedures by pointing to the hundreds of millions of these procedures that have been performed over the last 50 years. That argument cannot bear logical scrutiny. Tens of trillions of cigarettes have been purchased and smoked in the United States during the same time period. Does that prove that inhaling cigarette smoke is actually safe?

[His] hand-washing protocol was so vehemently opposed that the rejection by his peers literally drove him crazy.

For decades the tobacco industry argued that there was no legitimate, scientifically proven link between tobacco smoking and disease. Actually, the industry was technically right on this point.

Large population studies demonstrate that those who smoke cigarettes have a much higher incidence of lung cancer and heart disease than those who don't. But how do we know these observations are not coincidental or that there weren't other factors involved? After all, not everyone who inhales cigarette smoke, regardless of the quantity and length of time they do so, will get cancer or develop heart disease. It's also true that a total avoidance of tobacco smoke doesn't guarantee a life free from cancer or heart disease.

Then there's the clever but totally invalid "if cigarette smoking is so bad and so prevalent, why don't we see people dropping dead all around us from smoking-related disease?" The unstated "reasoning" behind this question is better stated like this:

- ✓ People all around us smoke cigarettes
- ✓ We never see smokers around us drop dead
- ✓ Therefore cigarette smoking is safe

However, at the end of these silly word games one would be hard pressed to find a single reasonable scientist on the planet who would claim cigarette smoking is free from serious health risks. That's why every pack of cigarettes sold in America comes with a bold admonition: "WARNING: cigarette smoking may be hazardous to your health."

In like manner, it is not valid to argue that root canal treatments are safe based on the unproved assumption that most people who have root canal-treated teeth are not sick. It is also true that people who don't have root canal-treated teeth still get cancer, heart disease, diabetes, dementia, etc., but that argument does not prove or disprove the safety of the root canal procedure. And to argue otherwise is completely disingenuous and deliberately misleading at best.

By now, it should not be necessary to disprove this logical fallacy: "if root canal-treated teeth are so bad, why don't we see people dropping dead all around us?"

The only way to actually prove the safety of root canal treatments would be to conduct repeatable scientific studies. These studies would have to

1) Demonstrate that root canal-treated teeth are, in fact, pathogen- and toxin-free, or, "if" infected,

2) Show that such disease-causing agents in the teeth cannot leak into the bloodstream or lymphatic system around them.

Such studies have not been published or they would have been broadcast from the rooftops.

Small Technicality Hides Overwhelming Evidence

For 12 years we have contended that there is more than sufficient scientific evidence to link root canal-treated teeth and disease. Rather than admitting that the issue is worthy of honest investigation, however, opponents have countered, as recently as 2014, with generic statements like the following:

> In *1951*, the *Journal of the American Dental Association* took the extraordinary step of publishing a special edition *reviewing the scientific literature* and shifted the standard of practice back to endodontic treatment for teeth with non-vital pulp in instances where the tooth could be saved. The *JADA* reviewed Dr. Price's research techniques from the 1920s and noted that they *lacked many aspects of modern scientific research, including absence of proper*

control groups and induction of excessive doses of bacteria.[1] [emphasis added]

Dr. Weston Price, like Dr. Ignac Semmelweis, voiced concern about an accepted procedure that might be responsible for causing disease. Most root canal procedures are performed due to infection already inside the normally sterile pulp and root system within a tooth. Price questioned the accepted notion that current endodontic (root canal) treatment could successfully disinfect an admittedly infected tooth.

To confirm his theory, he conducted meticulous experiments on extracted root canal-treated teeth. In one case, he placed such a tooth under the skin of a rabbit. The rabbit died within four days. He removed the tooth and implanted it in another rabbit. It died quickly as well. Then he repeated this procedure with another 30 rabbits in succession. They all died within four days of subcutaneous placement.

Ultimately, Price would test thousands of teeth for infection and toxicity. His tests clearly demonstrated that:

✓ *All* extracted teeth previously subjected to root canal treatment still contained pathogenic microbes and toxins.

✓ *All* of the extracted root canal-treated teeth were impossible to disinfect, even with sterilization methods that cannot be employed while a tooth is still in the mouth.

✓ *All* of the 32 rabbits noted above died within 4 days after having the same extracted root canal-treated tooth placed directly under the skin.

✓ **None** of the rabbits that had a non-root canal-treated tooth implanted under the skin showed any ill effects.

These results so convinced Dr. Price of the toxic and infected nature of root canal-treated teeth, he postulated that such teeth, while still in the mouth of a patient, were likely seeding infections and disease in other parts of the body.

Admittedly, some took his theory too far. Some dentists and physicians declared open season on teeth—extracting even vital, non-infected teeth—presuming them to be at the root of virtually every disease. They began to indiscriminately extract all suspected teeth from their sick patients expecting an immediate cure. In some cases, cures were reported. In many others, no post-extraction improvements were seen.

Dental professionals have been quick to highlight this indiscriminate tooth extraction as a way to discredit the entire argument against root canal treatment. But we fail to see how pointing out the reckless, "tooth-jerk" response of some establishes the safety of a root canal-treated tooth. The *practice* of indiscriminate tooth extraction and the *safety* of root canal-treated teeth are totally unrelated.

Another common argument fails the logic test as well. Weston Price implanted thousands of extracted root canal-treated teeth under the skin of rabbits. Without exception, all these animals quickly died or developed the **same disease** as the patients from whom the teeth had been removed. None of the rabbits that had non-root canal-treated teeth implanted ever got sick.

No **honest** scientist on the planet, after reviewing the findings above, could declare the root canal procedure absolutely safe simply because the researcher failed to use a control protocol adopted after his death. Even if Dr. Price's techniques failed to meet current research standards, he presented enough damning evidence to justify further testing. Why didn't the American Dental Association sponsor such testing?

Why Such Efforts by the Dental Profession to Discount Even the Current Evidence?

In light of all the evidence showing the association of root canal-treated teeth to systemic disease, we were perplexed as to why the dental profession has continued to discount all this evidence. Setting aside the monetary incentive, there must be other reasons why the profession so aggressively attacks anybody who made this logical connection after reviewing all of the available data. Even if the ADA was not 100% convinced, shouldn't they at least be curious to launch new studies here in the United States instead of making the blanket statement that under no circumstances can a root canal-treated tooth cause or contribute to systemic disease?

Explain to any intelligent layperson who has no ideological ties to the dental profession the essence of what we are saying in this book, namely:

✓ That root canal-treated teeth are not sterile and can contain pathogenic bacteria,

   ✓ That these bacteria and their toxins can get out
      of the tooth and the associated apical periodon-
      titis found around most all root canal-treated
      teeth, and

   ✓ That in a subset of people these teeth can cause
      or contribute to systemic disease.

Cite a few studies supporting these statements and almost everybody will say that this makes total sense. They get it. No great leap of faith required. Make the same statements to most dentists and they will vehemently deny that this is true. Why the difference in acceptance between these two groups?

At first it may seem like the dentists should be better able to accept this statement as true when presented with all of the supporting studies. After all, dentists have the education and professional experience to fully understand the science. However, it is likely this very education and experience make it difficult or impossible to accept any evidence that contradicts the core ideology and the "group think" of the profession. It is much easier for a person with no stake in the game to objectively evaluate data and form a conclusion.

Probably the main reason that dentists continue to deny any systemic risk associated with root canal-treated teeth is because of confirmation bias. Confirmation bias is the acceptance of information that confirms a belief system while ignoring information that challenges that already accepted belief system.

This happens all the time in politics where each polit- ical party interprets the same set of objective facts in completely opposite ways. Just turn on the various cable news channels and this becomes quite obvious.

Consider the case of manned space exploration. What NASA accomplished from 1960-1972 with the Mercury, Gemini, and Apollo moon landing programs is simply amazing. It seemed that the attitude of most everyone involved with the space program at the time was one of extreme personal pride in their job. The thinking throughout NASA and all of the sub-contractors was "if a part was going to fail, it was not going to be my part."

But something changed within NASA over time. Maybe it was the ballooning bureaucracy or the political and economic pressures dictating policy. Regardless, the NASA that landed Neil Armstrong and Buzz Aldrin on the moon on Apollo 11 in 1969 was not the same NASA that ignored the problems with the solid rocket booster joints that caused the space shuttle Challenger accident, or the constant shedding of foam from the main fuel tank that damaged the wing of the space shuttle Columbia and caused it's destruction upon reentry. Let's look how confirmation bias led to these two tragic accidents.

The space shuttle Challenger, with a crew of seven astronauts, was about to lift off from Cape Canaveral on January 28, 1986. On previous missions engineers at Morton Thiokol, maker of the space shuttle solid rocket boosters, observed damage to the O-ring seals between segments of the solid rocket boosters. These O-rings sealed the joint between booster segments and were essential to prevent hot gases from leaking out from these joints. One these engineers, Roger Boisjoly, had sent memos to his superiors warning that cold temperatures would make these O-rings less flexible and impair their ability to seal the rocket segments. On the morning of the Challenger launch, temperatures were at the freezing mark and Boisjoly strongly advised that the launch be postponed until it got warmer. Morton Thiokol and NASA had discussions on the integrity of the O-rings and the consensus was that there had never been a catastrophic O-ring failure in the past and that O-ring damage had also occurred on flights when the weather was warmer. Allan McDonald, senior management representative for Morton Thiokol at the Kennedy Space Center, refused to give a launch recommendation believing that the solid rocket booster was not safe to launch at these cold temperatures. NASA ignored McDonald's no-go recommendation and went back to the Morton Thiokol plant in Utah who gave the go for launch. The decision was made to launch Challenger.

Seventy-two seconds after launch the main fuel tank exploded due to an intense flame escaping the failed joint seal in the solid rocket booster striking the main fuel tank. All seven astronauts on board were killed. The O-rings did fail. Boisjoly and McDonald were right. Yet in spite of all the evidence that cold weather can prevent the solid rocket booster segments from sealing properly, NASA launched anyway.

During the Rogers Commission investigation of this accident, Physics professor Dr. Richard Feynmann took a piece of O-ring material and demonstrated the flexibility and pliability of the O-ring at room temperature. He then put the piece of O-ring in a glass of ice water for a few minutes. When he removed it the O-ring was stiff and inflexible. Cold made this O-ring material less likely to seal the gap between the solid rocket booster segments. This very simple demonstration showed the obvious and what Boisjoly and McDonald had been stating all along.

Tragedy struck the space shuttle Columbia on February 1, 2003. Launched on January 16, 2003, a suitcase-sized piece of foam insulation broke off from the external fuel tank and struck the left wing of the space shuttle. Foam has broken off of the main fuel tank just about every space shuttle launch without incident so it was considered routine and safe to launch. Not this time. A piece of foam struck the left wing of the orbiter as the shuttle was accelerating to space and put a hole in the left wing. The shuttle was doomed. A breach of the heat shield tiles in this location proved catastrophic, as the hot gases during reentry entered the left wing causing it to fail. The shuttle broke apart over Texas killing all seven astronauts.

> *In spite of all the evidence that cold weather can prevent the solid rocket booster segments from sealing properly, NASA launched anyway.*

The Columbia Accident Investigation Board Report stated:

> Management decisions made during Columbia's final flight reflect missed opportunities, blocked or ineffective communications channels, flawed analysis, and ineffective leadership. Perhaps the most striking is the fact that management.... displayed no interest in understanding a problem and it's implications....In fact, their management techniques unknowingly imposed barriers

that kept at bay both engineering concerns and dissenting views, and ultimately helped create "blind spots" that prevented them from seeing the danger the foam strike posed.

If confirmation bias can happen to the rocket scientists at NASA, it can certainly happen within the ADA. We will discuss the systemic risks of root canal-treated teeth and present the research supporting our assertions, and leave it up to the reader to draw their own logical conclusions. As noted by two Stanford psychologists:

> Beliefs can survive potent logical or empirical challenges. They can survive and even be bolstered by evidence that the most uncommitted observers would agree demands some weakening of such beliefs. They can even survive the total destruction of their original evidential basis.[1]

Who Should Bear the Burden of Proof?

Instead, proponents continue to make an unchallenged and unequivocal claim that "root canal treatment is safe." Rather than conduct their own studies, they rely on self-serving reviews and committee conclusions that dismiss Price's work based on technicalities. Poking holes in his research techniques cannot hide the gaping absence of research demonstrating the safety of root canal-treated teeth.

Since such research is unlikely to be undertaken in the near future, if ever, the goal of this book is to present a large body of steadily growing scientific evidence showing that:

1) Disease in one part of the body [called a focal infection] can and does produce disease in another part of the body, even when the infection at the original source is not clinically evident [the focus].

2) Nearly all, if not all, root canal-treated teeth are chronically infected.

3) It is impossible with current techniques to remove all pathogenic microorganisms from an infected root canal-treated tooth.

4) Apical periodontitis (an infection of the tissues around the root tip of the tooth) originates from teeth with an infected pulp, or root canal space.

5) Recent studies link apical periodontitis to a host of other diseases in organs and structures throughout the body, sparing no organs or tissues.

6) The immune system does not and cannot provide reliable protection against any and all pathogens and associated toxins originating from apical periodontitis or the infected tooth from whence it came.

7) The mere presence of root canal-treated teeth has been clinically associated with the increased risk of heart disease.

8) Populations of pathogenic organisms that are normally found only in infected teeth have been found in the diseased organ tissues of patients with root canal-treated teeth.

The American Association of Endodontists official website states: "There is no valid, scientific evidence
linking root canal-treated teeth and disease elsewhere
in the body." Contrary to that claim, we contend that the
volume of scientific research listed above and presented
throughout this book is more than sufficient to demonstrate a connection, and likely cause-and-effect relationship, between root canal-treated teeth and a wide array of
diseases.

Finally, we will present safer alternatives to the
uniformly futile approaches that try to disinfect a tooth
infected by the root canal procedure.

Examine the evidence presented herein. Study
the counterarguments from root canal advocates. At a
minimum, we're confident that even the most confirmed
skeptic who maintains an open mind will agree that there
is reason to doubt the safety of the root canal procedure.

Ultimately, as in the case of Semmelweis and hand-
washing, we still believe that legitimate scientific research,
if undertaken, will validate our claim. It is our hope that by
expanding upon the information we first published in 2002
we will inspire both the dental and medical professions to
actively research this subject and empower you, the reader
and the patient, to intelligently and appropriately question
your dentist about the risk and benefit of all your treatment
options.

Robert Kulacz, DDS and Thomas E. Levy, MD, JD

CHAPTER ONE

THE CASE *Against Root Canal Treatment*

Endangering the Body to "Save Your Smile"

According to the official website of the American Association of Endodontists, the goal of a root canal treatment is to "relieve your tooth pain and save your smile." The same website goes on to explain the procedure:

> "Endodontic [root canal] treatment treats the inside of the tooth. Endodontic treatment is necessary when the pulp becomes inflamed or infected. The inflammation or infection can have a variety of causes: deep decay, repeated dental procedures on the tooth, faulty crowns, or a crack or chip in the tooth. In addition, trauma to a tooth may cause pulp damage even if the tooth has no visible chips or cracks. If pulp inflammation or infection is left untreated, it can cause pain or lead to an abscess. "

"How does endodontic treatment save the tooth?
During root canal treatment, the inflamed or
infected pulp is removed and the inside of the
tooth is carefully cleaned and disinfected, then
filled and sealed with a rubber-like material called
gutta-percha. Afterwards, the tooth is restored
with a crown or filling for protection. After restoration, the tooth continues to function like any
other tooth."[1]

The goal seems noble and innocent enough. It's all good, right?

On the face of it, a tooth has been "saved," but
there's a devil in the details. A previously infected
tooth that now maintains a beautiful smile and is
without pain, in their words "saved," does not mean
that the tooth is necessarily safe. Overwhelming
scientific evidence shows that virtually all root canal-treated teeth are still infected and slowly and
continually leak disease-causing pathogens and
toxins into the rest of the body as long as they remain in the mouth.

Removing the pain-sensing nerves from a tooth
and blocking all access to the infection-fighting immune system does not "cure" the tooth any more
than a local anesthetic "cures" a painful boil. The
pain has been resolved, but nothing has been done
to cure the underlying infection. Ignorance may be

bliss... until a stroke, heart attack, dementia, arthritis, or cancer shatters the blissful calm.

Based on the data that is being collected and published now, the health impact of root canal-treated teeth is staggering. According to industry statistics, over 25 million root canal procedures (endodontic treatments) are performed in the United States every year. Recent research would indicate that the secondary health cost as a result of these procedures is many times greater than the cost of the procedures themselves. And, of course,

Removing the pain-sensing nerves from a tooth and blocking all access to the infection-fighting immune system does not "cure" the tooth.

that's only the financial impact of these procedures. The human price is much steeper.

It should be understood from the beginning that it is the root canal treatment procedure, and this treatment alone, that is being brought into question. Nothing in this book is intended to state or imply malpractice or intended harm by those who perform this treatment. The vast majority of these professionals are sincere, hard-working, conscientious, and very interested in the health of their patients. These men and women are only doing what they have been taught to do. They are simply doing a pro-

cedure they believe to be beneficial, and they are asserting what they have been taught to believe.

On the other hand, materials and websites that
promote endodontic treatment often claim that
there are no scientific grounds for concern about the
safety of such therapies. That is simply not true, and
it is grossly irresponsible. Recent scientific evidence
will be presented to show that the infection and
toxins that remain in virtually all root canal-treated
teeth are intimately linked with

✓ Alzheimer's disease (onset/progression)
✓ Ankylosing spondylitis
✓ Asthma (worsening and increased bronchial
   inflammation)
✓ Birth problems (low birth weights, prema-
   ture birth, lower maternal hemoglobin
   levels)
✓ Cancer (of the lung, kidney, pancreas, and
   blood)
✓ Cardiac calcification
✓ Cerebrovascular disease
✓ Chronic obstructive pulmonary disease
   (COPD) and its worsening
✓ Coronary heart disease (CHD)
✓ Diabetes
✓ Endothelial dysfunction
✓ Epilepsy (increased seizure severity)

✓ Hearing loss (sudden sensorineural)
✓ High blood pressure (hypertension and increased mortality from hypertension)
✓ Increased serum cholesterol and LDL levels
✓ Inflammatory bowel disease
✓ Kidney disease
✓ Metabolic syndrome (leading to increased CHD)
✓ Obesity
✓ Osteoporosis (stimulation of osteoclastic activity)
✓ Pneumonia and other lung infections
✓ Preeclampsia (increased risk)
✓ Psoriasis
✓ Rheumatoid arthritis
✓ Septic pulmonary embolism
✓ Stroke (increased risk and greater neurological deficit)
✓ Systemic lupus erythematosus and its worsening
✓ Vascular disease (such as Buerger's disease and varicose veins)
✓ Critical vitamin deficiencies (C and D)

Additionally, anatomical evidence will show that the goal of root canal treatment, namely to "save" the tooth by removing the infection (sterilization) and to create a bacteria-tight seal to prevent re-infection and leakage, is essentially impossible in both theory and execution. In the coming chapters scientific studies will be used to demonstrate that virtually all root canal-treated teeth are, in fact, infected and leaking.

Endodontic proponents assert that the healthy immune system is capable of handling any infectious bacteria remaining after the root canal treatment in a matter of minutes.

Endodontic proponents assert that the healthy immune system is capable of handling any infectious bacteria remaining after the root canal treatment in a matter of minutes. The fallacy of this notion will be fully exposed with scientific examples and precedent. Unfortunately, it's not just pathogens that present the danger. The microbes in the oxygen-starved environment of a root canal-treated tooth produce exotoxins that are biologically highly toxic and virtually untouchable by the immune system.

Some have questioned the actual danger of endodontic treatment simply by noting that if the claims were true, people would be falling dead all around us from root canal-treated teeth.

The reality is that millions *are* dying from heart disease, kidney disease, diabetes, cancer, and dementia. Many others *are* suffering with arthritis, obesity, metabolic syndrome, and high blood pressure. And in those cases where root canal-treated teeth have been the cause of the death and suffering, the typically pain-free treated teeth just sit in the mouth quietly exporting their pathogens and toxins—day after day, year after year—often with little or no sign of harmful activity unless actively investigated with clinical evaluation and laboratory testing.

*The reality is that millions **are** dying from heart disease, kidney disease, diabetes, cancer, and dementia. Many others **are** suffering with arthritis, obesity, metabolic syndrome, and high blood pressure.*

For sure, not all who are dying or suffering are doing so because of root canal-treated teeth. But current evidence says some people certainly are. Root canal-treated teeth increase the risk of disease, period. Few are acknowledging this risk.

Serious warnings are in order. Patients must be informed of the documented risks of root canal treatment and offered the alternatives to root canal procedures. Simply put, there must be a full informed consent offered patients contemplating this procedure. Dentists cannot selectively omit peer-reviewed published research data describing the systemic health risks of root canal-treated teeth in talking with patients while assuring them that the root canal treatment is a completely harmless procedure. The chapters ahead present the evidence, sound the warning, state the risks, and present the alternatives.

CHAPTER TWO

OBJECTIVE *of Root Canal Treatment*

Mission Impossible?

The stated goal of endodontic therapy (a root canal procedure) is to "save" an infected tooth. In more technical terms it is an attempt to preserve the external structure and function of the tooth by extracting the infected tissues in the middle of the tooth. Once the diseased pulp tissue, the nerves, and the blood supply have been removed, the internal surfaces of the pulp cavity are widened and shaped with special instruments.

During the root canal treatment, disinfectant chemicals are introduced into the root canal system in an attempt to destroy any infection. Ultimately, the evacuated cavity is filled and sealed as best as possible to minimize re-infection. In the vast majority of cases, the pain is gone with little visible change to the external structure of the tooth and with no loss of chewing function. Admittedly, these are all positive outcomes and worthy goals, but they do not address the indwelling chronic infection that remains in the vast majority of such treated teeth.

Two membership organizations, the American Dental Association (ADA) and the American Association of Endodontists (AAE), fervently defend the safety and effectiveness of root canal therapy. In their promotion of root canal therapy, these associations and their members point to impressive statistics that suggest a high success rate. They also claim that there is "no science" to justify concerns about the procedure's safety.

These organizations, whose primary role is to protect and defend member interests, also accuse detractors of recycling "urban legends" that were supposedly debunked over 60 years ago. Careful review of the scientific literature shows that these urban legends may not be urban legends at all, and it calls into serious question their definitive claim that root canal-treated teeth pose absolutely no risk to systemic health.

The touted success rate (some claim a figure as high as 97%) is impressive until the method of arriving at their definition of "success" is revealed. If a root canal-treated tooth simply survives eight years in the mouth without external signs of infection, the procedure is deemed a success.[1] It doesn't matter what new health problems might have developed during that time.

In reality, the mere presence of an intact root canal-treated tooth does not guarantee that it is not harboring infection any more than it guarantees that a perfectly intact can of tomatoes is not tainted with botulism. Remember, the nerves inside the root canal-treated tooth that would have normally signaled infection have been removed.

Root canal treatment does more to the tooth than alleviate pain while preserving external appearance and chewing function. Root canal therapy totally disconnects the tooth's injury and infection detection system—the tooth is essentially incapable of fighting pathogens. The blood and lymphatic "supply lines" that deliver vital nutrients, oxygen, antibodies, immune cells, antioxidants, and all other elements employed by the body to stay healthy have been totally removed. In other words, without access to the immune system, there can be no immune response to infection.

> *Root canal therapy totally disconnects the tooth's injury and infection detection system.*

Therefore, any infection within the root canal-treated tooth will remain in the tooth without any visible signs of infection such as inflammation, pus, or swelling.

Is it possible that root canal therapy inadvertently establishes a safe harbor for microorganisms that could subsequently promote disease in other parts of the body? Early researchers warned that this was so and now current research is validating their concerns.

During the last decade significant and growing research shows that root canal therapy fails to sterilize teeth with alarming frequency. Other research demonstrates that current filling and sealing methods *routinely* fail to effectively seal a root canal-treated tooth. The most powerful indictment comes from several recent studies that demonstrate a consistent link between a host of diseases and root canal-treated teeth.

Almost 90 years ago, Weston Price, Frank Billings, Edward Rosenow, and others published volumes of research that warned of serious health dangers associated with root canal-treated teeth. Root canal therapy proponents claim that these concerns were debunked in a special edition of the *Journal of the American Dental Association* (*JADA*) that was published over 60 years ago.[2]

Recent discoveries suggest that self-interest may have blinded those who claimed to have "debunked" the earlier research. In the last 20 years, many studies have tied root canal therapy to increased risks for cancer, heart disease, diabetes, dementia, and other diseases.

These connections are frighteningly similar to those reported by Price, Billings, and Rosenow. At a bare minimum, these new studies justify a close reevaluation of the initial research. They also cry out for some definitive ways to verify an infection-free, toxin-free, and safely-sealed state of root canal-treated teeth, if indeed such a state is physiologically and anatomically possible with current root canal procedures.

These studies, both new and old, provide "smoking gun" evidence against root canal treatment that will be discussed at length in Chapter Five. The primary purpose of this chapter is to show the nearly insurmountable challenges faced by every root canal therapist. Initial obstacles spring from the realities of tooth anatomy. Other challenges come from the limitations in the instruments, materials, and technical aspects of the procedure itself.

The Daunting Anatomy of a Tooth

To gain any appreciation of the challenges standing in the way of a technically successful root canal procedure, it is important to have a basic understanding of tooth anatomy (Figure 2-1). Each tooth is anchored in the jawbone by one or more roots. A front tooth usually has one root, and a larger back tooth (molar), can have as many as three or four roots. Each of the roots has a nerve supply and a blood vessel supply, and these enter the bottom of the root from the jawbone. These nerves and blood vessels extend up the root into an area called the pulp chamber. Dental pulp (Figure 2-1) is a loose connective tissue that contains a complex assortment of cell types and substances. It is not necessary for the reader know what all these

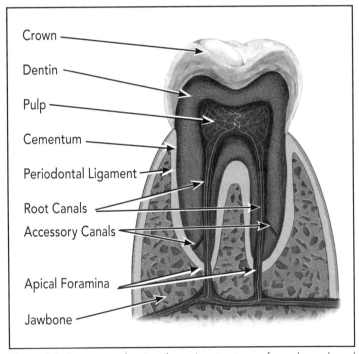

Crown
Dentin
Pulp
Cementum
Periodontal Ligament
Root Canals
Accessory Canals
Apical Foramina
Jawbone

Figure 2-1: A cut-away showing the major structures of a molar anchored in the jawbone.

components are or what they do to appreciate the challenges of the procedure, but a summary review of them provides a small appreciation for the valuable contents that are being extracted from the tooth. Those components include:

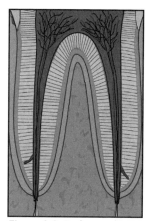

Figure 2-2: Dark area shows pulp extending from the pulp chamber to the root canals and accessory canals branching off each root canal.

- ✓ A variety of immune and structural cells, including fibroblasts and undifferentiated mesenchymal cells, as well as macrophages, lymphocytes, histiocytes, granulocytes, mast cells, and plasma cells required for the maintenance and defense of the tissue.
- ✓ Fibrous matrix, largely composed of type I and II collagen fibers.
- ✓ Ground substance, which is the environment that surrounds both cells and fibers of the pulp and is rich in proteoglycans, glycoproteins, and water.
- ✓ Perivascular cells, which are important, undifferentiated mesenchymal cells within the pulp that facilitate the recruitment of newly differentiated cells to replace others

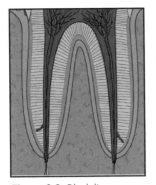

Figure 2-3: Black lines represent the nerves and blood vessels extending out of the apical foramen at the tip of each root.

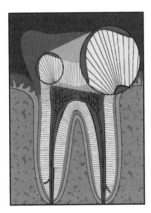

Figure 2-4: Lightest area shows dentin surrounding the pulp chamber and root canal with an inset showing the dentinal tubules radiating outward.

when they are lost, namely odontoblasts.

✓ Odontoblasts, the cells that comprise the outermost layer of the pulp, immediately adjacent to the dentin component of the tooth. These cells are responsible for the secretion of dentin and the formation of dentinal tubules in the crown and root areas.

The pulp is complex enough that many call it an organ, and it is this part of the tooth that the root canal procedure attempts to completely remove.

With the exception of the opening at the tip of each root (apical foramen), the pulp chamber is completely encased by dentin. One or more accessory canals (Figure 2-2) often branch from each root canal while the blood vessels and nerves pass out of the tooth through the apical foramen (Figure 2-3) near the tip of each root.

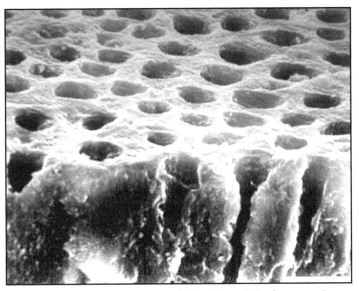

Figure 2-5: Photograph of dentinal tubules. If the tubules from a single tooth were placed end-to-end, it would extend up to 3 miles. There are from 5,000 to 90,000 tubules per square millimeter (about the size of this little square ▪). The sectioned tubules in the front of this photograph show how easily bacteria could hide in them, safe from mechanical, laser, and even chemical eradication.

Photo courtesy of Royal Society Publishing
Reproduced from a study on the parametric effect of phase anisotropy on the micromechanical behavior of dentin adhesive interfaces.[3]

Dentin (Figure 2-4) makes up the bulk of the tooth's hard tissue. Although firm and rigid, the dentin is not solid. It is filled with microscopic tubules (Figure 2-5) that radiate from the pulp, through the entire thickness of the dentin. If the dentinal tubules from a single tooth were placed end-to-end they would extend up to three miles in length. One of the functions of the dentinal tubules is the signaling of temperature and

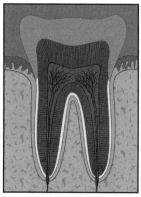

Figure 2-6: White outline shows the cementum layer that encapsulates the dentin.

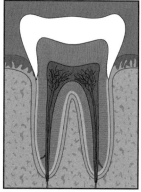

Figure 2-7: White area shows the crown of the tooth.

pressure changes occurring on the outside of the tooth to the nerves in the pulp as part of the tooth's injury and infection warning system.

The dentin component of the tooth root is completely encased, again with the exception of the apical foramen, by a thin shell called cementum (Figure 2-6).

The top portion, or the crown (Figure 2-7) of each tooth is covered with enamel. In most cases, while the tooth remains in the mouth, the crown is the only visible part of a tooth.

The stereotypical drawings shown here are helpful but fail to illustrate one of the major complicating factors of any root canal procedure. Like fingerprints, all teeth are incredibly unique. Visible variances in the size, the color, the number of roots, and the overall shape only begin to hint at the significant variations inside each tooth.

Typically, each tooth root contains from one to four canals, and each canal can have any of a variety

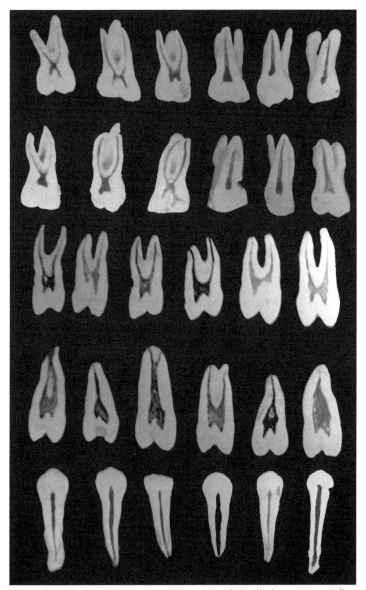

Figure 2-8: The immense variations in root canal morphology— especially the number and shape of root canals — presents a great challenge for the dentist attempting to sterilize, fill, and seal a tooth.

Photo collage compiled from Grossman's *Root Canal Therapy* textbook

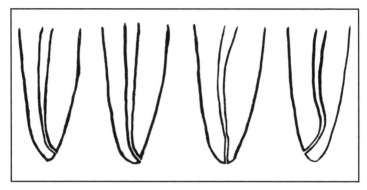

Figure 2-9: As the root canal travels from the pulp chamber to the apex of the root, it can take a number of different twists and turns. This adds to the challenge of pulp removal, sterilization, filling, and sealing an infected tooth.
Drawing from Grossman's *Root Canal Therapy* textbook

of shapes and sizes. To complicate the challenge, many of these internal variations are invisible on an X-ray or through the opening in the top of the tooth that is created by the dentist in order to perform the root canal procedure.

The main canals can even have branches and fork into two sections making cleaning difficult or impossible. Figure 2-8 is a photograph that gives a small indication of the variety of shapes and sizes, inside and out, of teeth. Figure 2-9 is a drawing that depicts the interesting twists and turns that can appear at the tip (apex) of the tooth root.

The endodontist's mission, then, is to:

✓ Drill a sizable entry point in the tooth to expose the pulp cavity. For premolars and molars this will be in the top of the crown, and for front teeth, in the back. *This is readily achieved.*

✓ Remove all of the pulp and infected tissues within the pulp chamber. *This is readily achieved.*

✓ Thoroughly clean, shape, and widen all of the separate tooth roots, which can number from one to four or more for each tooth, may be curved in numerous directions, and are the diameter of a pencil lead or smaller. Although the main canal system may be thoroughly cleaned by a skilled practitioner, the numerous accessory canals that branch off the main canals cannot be reached and cleaned. Dentists rely on irrigation to clean these accessory canals with only limited success. *This step is never completely achieved.*

✓ Since ALL the infection needs to be removed, the miles of dentinal tubules that routinely harbor bacteria when the pulp is infected should be scrubbed clean even though these tubules cannot be seen without the aid of a microscope. (This step is mechanically impossible, so the endodontist must rely upon a chemical disinfectant to kill all microorganisms. The challenge of disinfecting a tooth is covered in the next section.) *This is never achieved.*

✓ In some teeth, especially the upper first molars, there are small canals that cannot easily be seen. If these canals are missed during the root canal procedure they will not be cleaned at all and will still contain necrotic (dead) and infected tissue.

✓ If the mission fails to remove all infected tissues and all pathogens, by definition the tooth is still infected, even if the tooth is filled and sealed.

Hasn't modern science developed high-tech instruments and techniques that can accomplish this procedure? It is true that efforts have been made to improve instruments and materials over the years. However, despite the "improvements" introduced in the last couple of decades, researchers in recent studies still judge a majority of root canal-treated teeth as "failures" simply on the basis of visible observation. These studies will be discussed in Chapter Three.

If the mission fails to remove all infected tissues and all pathogens, by definition the tooth is still infected.

The Challenges of Disinfecting a Root Canal-Treated Tooth

Endodontists now actually acknowledge the impossibility of physically removing all infection and pathogens from the tooth, but they confidently rely on the power of disinfectant agents to finish the job. Admittedly, these disinfectants are powerful and are capable of handling all the microbes that they actually touch.

However, the physical and biological laws that these chemicals must overcome are virtually insurmountable. Imagine a handful of small-diameter straws (like coffee stirrers) lying in a large dish filled with beaten raw eggs that are infected with salmonella. After three or four hours, remove the straws from the egg mixture and let them sit for a day or two. One by one, close one end of a straw with your index finger and dip it into a pan filled with lukewarm water and some liquid chlorine bleach. Without agitating the straw, hold it under the water for about three minutes, remove, and let it air dry. Repeat with each straw.

What is the possibility that all these straws are now free from salmonella? Based on published sanitation standards the appropriate exposure time and temperature of the bleach solution will kill salmonella. But there remains a major hurdle. The

standards require a thorough cleaning, including removal of food and other debris, prior to sanitizing.
Also, the microbes are only killed if they come in
direct contact with the disinfec-

*Considering
the visual,
physical, and
environmental
obstacles, the
changes of fully
sterilizing a tooth
are impossible,
both in theory and
in practice.*

tant. Since each straw contains
globs and clots of dried egg, and
since the disinfectant cannot
flow through the entire length of
the straw, a significant population of bacteria would *always* be
expected to remain and grow in
each straw. And finally, sanitation experts further concede that
even in a place where all the surfaces can be thoroughly washed
and exposed to a disinfectant for
sufficient time, a few bacteria will always remain,
allowing for new growth.[4]

Compared to the straw example, the sterilization challenges in a tooth are mind-boggling. The
dentinal tubules are very tiny and there are many
millions of them.[5] Like the straws, they have not
been cleared of infected matter and dentinal fluid.
Additionally, they are covered by cementum, which
severely limits penetration of the disinfectant into
each tubule in the tooth. Considering the visual,
physical, and environmental obstacles, it is impos-

sible to fully sterilize a tooth, both in theory and in practice.

Thankfully, one does not have to rely on imagination, theory, probabilities, or even blind faith to grasp the impossibility of sterilizing a root canal-treated tooth. Research has shown that sterilizing an *extracted* tooth is nearly impossible, even when employing chemicals that could never be used while a tooth was in someone's mouth. Other recent studies that will be discussed in the next chapter also show that all root canal-treated teeth are and will remain infected.

Even a tiny population of bacteria or fungi that survives in a missed canal or somewhere in the miles of dentinal tubules can multiply into a large colony. This would be especially true when these microorganisms are left in a dark, warm, moist place, with organic material like that found inside the dentin and unfilled pockets in a root canal-treated tooth. What's more, this perfect environment has been disconnected from the body's immune and infection warning systems, so they can be free to grow without immune system challenge or detection.

But, perhaps this is much ado about nothing. After all, millions upon millions of people have undergone root canal therapy on one or more teeth, most of those teeth are still in place and show no "infection" after eight years, and the average human lifespan is actually going up. So what's the big deal?

It could be similarly argued that millions upon millions of people have smoked cigarettes, the vast majority of them were still alive after eight years of habitual smoking with no signs of a problem, and the average lifespan has been going up since the turn of the 20th century—even during the time of greatest cigarette use. This kind of flawed logic could be used to justify many harmful activities.

While many may now concede that the root canal-treated tooth cannot be totally sterilized, the dental profession might offer the argument that a tiny colony of germs trapped in a tooth is not really a problem. This could be the case if the tooth had normal blood and fluid flow, with full access by a normally-functioning immune system. How can one know that these pathogens and their toxins are "trapped" or sealed within the root canal-treated tooth?

The Challenges of Sealing a Root Canal-Treated Tooth

When a dentist performs a root canal procedure on an infected tooth, the infected nerves, blood vessels, and connective tissue are cleaned from the pulp chamber and the main canal space as completely as possible. Then the primary canals are shaped and widened.

Once the endodontist determines that the cavity is sufficiently prepared, the process of filling it begins. Most commonly, a plant-based, rubber-like material called gutta-percha, along with a sealer, is used to fill and seal the root canal space. When the root canal space is deemed to be full, a temporary crown or filling is placed. Mission accomplished.

But how does the endodontist know there aren't any leaks? There are simple tests for checking the seals in a myriad of other situations. One can check the airtight seal on a bicycle inner tube by submerging the inflated tube in water. If no air bubbles appear around the tube, it's sealed. Plumbers check for leaks around joints by checking for wetness. Those who can their own food check for an indentation in the lid to verify that the jar is vacuum-sealed.

*Bacteria... leaked out of 80% of the teeth filled with gutta-percha **regardless** of which sealer was used.*

What does the endodontist do? He can check a post-procedure X-ray to verify that there are no large gaps without filling material, and that apex has not been overfilled. However, the resolution on X-rays are incapable of detecting any of the microscopic pockets big enough to harbor millions of pathogens. Nor can X-rays detect the tiny breaches in the seal that would permit bacteria or their toxins to seep out or that give access for pathogens to re-enter the tooth.

In the vast majority of cases it is just assumed that the tooth is sealed. Only the most blatant of failures would ever be detected by the methods currently employed. Assurance of success is usually based on visual confirmation that the gutta-percha fills up, and is flush with, the opening in the tooth, and on X-rays that show the gutta-percha extends approximately as far as the apical foramina.

Bacteria... were detected in 84% of the gutta-percha filled and sealed teeth after only 72 hours.

Research proves this root-filling method to be insufficient. A recent study tested different sealing agents by performing root canal treatments in extracted teeth. The researchers found that bacteria (*Streptococcus mutans*) leaked out of 80% of the teeth filled with gutta-percha **regardless** of which sealer was used. The same test using Resilon as the filler and Epiphany as the sealer had a bacterial leakage rate of 60%. These failures were seen within the first hour after sealing the teeth.[6]

In a similar test, bacteria (*Enterococcus faecalis*) were detected in 84% of the gutta-percha-filled and sealed teeth after only 72 hours.[7] Both these tests were conducted *in vitro* (outside the body). The failure rate on a tooth in a mouth would be expected to be even higher than that seen in the laboratory.

Desperately Seeking Sterility with Laser Technology

Lasers have already done many fantastic things and undoubtedly will continue to have even more impressive applications over time in all areas of science, including medicine and dentistry. Because of the vast utilization of this technology, lasers are often viewed as a treatment modality with unlimited potential. However, a laser works according to scientific principles, and there are straightforward, unchangeable reasons why it can never sterilize a root canal-treated tooth.

The power of a laser is in its ability to sharply focus light to make all the light waves travel in the same direction. Unlike a flashlight that scatters and diffuses light, laser light travels in a very thin straight line with very little dissipation or scatter over distance.

Herein lies the problem of using a laser for disinfecting a tooth. The inherent straightness of laser light is directly incompatible with the innately curved and multifaceted configuration of a tooth pulp. A laser is absolutely incapable of following any curve at all, whether in the primary canal or in any accessory canals or in the dentinal tubules. In like manner, laser light cannot bend in order to enter the lateral accessory canal branches or the tubules in the dentin.

A laser is absolutely incapable of following any curve at all; whether in the primary canal or any of the adjoining root canals.

A laser beam cannot kill a microorganism unless it shines directly on it. Therefore, it is absolutely impossible to insert a laser into the main canal of a pulp-evacuated tooth and expect it to kill the bacteria in all of the accessory canals or the dentinal tubules. Similarly, since the laser light cannot reach the periodontal ligament or the bone at the apex of the tooth, it is unable to kill the bacteria in those tissues as well. Bacteria would then rapidly re-infect the tooth even if, for the sake of argument, the laser did kill everything before that point.

Some dentists believe that the laser is sterilizing the entire tooth because they see the aiming laser light shining "through" the tooth. What they are in fact seeing is the glow emanating from around the tubular laser conduit and its tip, as well as the reflected and refracted light. This scattered, laser-associated light makes the entire tooth "glow" but it cannot carry the energy necessary to accomplish anything beyond that glow. It is the very nature of light to continue to bounce off reflective surfaces and be bent and transmitted through refractive surfaces. But once any reflection or refraction has occurred, the concentrated, microbe-killing effects of the original laser light have been lost.

To test this concept, an extracted tooth was given a complete root canal procedure with the cleaning and shaping of the canal performed exactly as would be done in the mouth. Dental plaque samples, which contain live bacteria, were then placed on the outside root surface for the full length of this treated tooth. The tooth was then treated with a dental laser that was set on 15 watts (this is significantly more energy than would be used on an actual tooth inside the mouth). Furthermore, this laser treatment was extended for roughly ten times the recommended exposure time. This

Laser treatment vastly more intense than is typically administered in the mouth... Areas "lit up" by reflected laser light showed no sterilization effect.

translates to a laser treatment vastly more intense than is typically administered in the mouth. The plaque samples were then retrieved for examination under a microscope.

If the laser had effectively sterilized the tooth, then no live bacteria should be present. Instead, microscopic examination revealed a host of bacteria that were very much alive. It appeared that the laser had no detectable effect on these plaque-associated bacteria. The laser was only able to sterilize that part of the tooth that was directly in front of the laser beam. Areas "lit up" by reflected and refracted laser light showed no sterilization effect, anymore than if they had been illuminated by a desk lamp.

Desperately Seeking Success with New Filling/Sealing Materials

The known deficiencies of gutta-percha as a filling/sealing agent have given rise to a couple of alternatives. The aforementioned Resilon, although outperforming gutta-percha in a leakage test, still failed in 60% of the teeth treated within one hour.

The other alternative that had some popularity in the past is Biocalex. Biocalex is a calcium oxide paste that converts to calcium carbonate in the evacuated root canal space. Proponents of Biocalex claim that it seeks out moisture in the tooth and expands somewhat into the lateral canals and dentinal tubules, thereby preventing leakage. Furthermore, the pH of Biocalex is very high meaning that it is very alkaline. This alkaline pH also helps to inhibit the growth of bacteria.

These properties of Biocalex would appear to be very desirable, and Biocalex would appear to be a better root canal filling material than gutta-percha.

However, the ability of Biocalex to completely seal off the main canal and inhibit bacterial growth still does not reconcile with the clinical and laboratory findings of individuals with Biocalex-filled root canal-treated teeth. Like gutta-percha-filled root canal spaces, Biocalex-filled teeth have also proved to be

Resilon, although outperforming gutta-percha in a leakage test, still failed in 60% of the teeth treated within one hour.

highly toxic on the Haley toxicity test for enzyme inhibition upon extraction, to be discussed in Chapter Three.

Just as would be expected in a typical root canal-treated tooth filled with gutta-percha, these extracted teeth that had been filled with Biocalex also demonstrate chronic osteomyelitis of the surrounding bone on pathology reports. Chronic osteomyelitis is inflamed bone that is nearly always infected. This would indicate that Biocalex does not make the tooth non-toxic and it does not prevent the infection of supporting bone.

There is also another important concern that is unique to the root canal-treated tooth filled with Biocalex. Root canal-treated teeth filled with gutta-percha classically have a very characteristic, easy-to-identify appearance on X-ray. There are an increasing number of people today who seek to have their root canal-treated teeth extracted in order to lessen their toxin exposure and hopefully improve their medical conditions. Biocalex has the added disadvantage of being very difficult, if not impossible, to be routinely identified on an X-ray unless the tooth has had another substance added to it to make it more visible on X-ray. Root canal spaces filled with gutta-percha, however, show up very prominently on X-ray.

Hopefully, a substance will eventually be developed to negate the toxicity of a root canal-treated tooth. Resilon and Biocalex definitely do not meet that need.

The Poor Prognosis for a Root Canal-Treated Tooth

Since the current materials used to fill evacuated root canal spaces do not make a perfect seal, there are two very serious implications:

✓ Even if a root canal-treated tooth were free from infection at the end of the procedure, the tooth will readily become infected.

✓ The infection in the root canal-treated tooth can always be expected to leak.

This leakage allows bacteria and their toxins access to the bloodstream with subsequent dissemination to the rest of the body. The filling materials used to seal an evacuated root canal space usually shrink away from the walls of the canal after placement, setting, and cooling, assuring an incomplete filling of that space. This consistently sets the stage for re-infection and leakage.

One other important point needs to be made concerning the ongoing quest to find a way to sterilize a root canal-treated tooth. Even if a technology could be found that could truly eradicate all of the bacteria in a root canal-treated tooth's root system, dentinal tubules, periodontal ligament, and surrounding infected bone and socket structures, the resulting sterile state would only be very short-lived.

As discussed previously, the root canal procedure destroys the internal connective tissue structure, nerve supply, and blood supply of the tooth, effectively blocking immune system function in the core of that tooth by blocking immune system access. When immune access is impeded in this fashion, bacteria are free to be reintroduced into the tooth and to re-colonize the tooth in fairly short order.

The mouth has an incredible abundance of microorganisms in it, and without an intact immune system with good access to all parts of the dead and non-viable root canal-treated tooth, core infection becomes quickly re-established.

On the basis of the challenges mentioned above due to complex tooth anatomy, the impossibility of sterilizing a tooth, and the difficulties of sealing a root canal-treated tooth, the prognosis is that all root canal-treated teeth are infected and leak. Is this a problem? Can't the immune system handle this, and how might this affect overall health? These are questions that will be addressed in the next three chapters.

CHAPTER THREE

EVALUATION *of Root Canal Treatment*

Massive Mission Failures

Every time a dentist or endodontist analyzes an X-ray of a visually stable root canal-treated tooth or examines such a tooth in a patient's mouth, his observations are expected to confirm the notion that all but a small number of root canal procedures are "successful." Of course, the dental school professors, textbooks, and patient literature all support this conclusion, yet the criteria by which these assumptions are made are fundamentally flawed.

Unfortunately, sole dependence on these two methods may provide a dangerously deceptive view of reality. X-rays are extremely helpful, and visual examination is necessary, but neither can accurately determine the presence or absence of pathogens inside the tooth. That's why medical doctors rely on blood tests and cultures to diagnose infection.

In the previous chapter the possibilities of performing a truly infection-free, perfectly-sealed root canal procedure were explored. These possibilities were evaluated against the backdrop of enormous anatomical and technical challenges that we believe really cannot be overcome. From that vantage point it was concluded that the infection-free goal of root canal treatment is simply impossible, both in practice and theory. If science can change this root canal procedure failing in the future, that would be great.

This chapter reviews what researchers have reported in the radiological and toxicological analysis of root canal-treated teeth.

The Criteria for Evaluating True Success

In the previous chapter a couple of *in vivo* root canal filling/sealing material studies were cited. These studies reported that the tested root canal sealing materials were unable to prevent leakage up to 80% of the time. Furthermore this leakage was evident within 1 to 72 hours after the procedure was performed.[1,2] So one way—but certainly not the only way—to evaluate the success of a root canal procedure would be to determine the frequency that such teeth are leaking as they sit in the mouths of patients.

A major evidence of microbial infection of the root canal-treated tooth is a condition known as apical periodontitis, also called a periapical lesion on X-ray. When a periapical lesion appears after a root canal procedure has been performed, it guarantees an infection in the tooth as well as a breach in the seal.

Frequently a dentist will detect apical periodontitis upon X-ray examination. X-rays cannot reveal actual infection, but because this condition can cause the partial resorption (dissolving) of bone tissue, a dark area outside the tip of the tooth root will result. When such a dark area beyond the tip of the tooth root is visible on an X-ray, it reliably indicates the presence of an infection.

When an infection is indicated on an X-ray it is certainly confirmation of it.

Detailed analysis shows that X-rays often miss infection that is present and frequently under-represent the extent of the infection that is actually present. At other times, no difference in appearance when compared to adjacent vital teeth was seen and X-rays failed to detect extensive infection that was found after extraction.[3] In other words, an X-ray can confirm infection but a negative X-ray never rules infection out.

There are several reasons why the presence of apical periodontitis may not appear on an X-ray. Even if resorption has taken place, it may not be detected because the missing bone can be obscured by another root of the same tooth or by a heavy mass of bone in front of or behind the darkened area. An infection may also escape detection because chronic infection and inflammation can sometimes initiate a reactive bone formation (condensing osteitis) rather than bone resorption.

Only 14% of the examined root canal-treated teeth were deemed to be adequate according to currently accepted standards.

The point is this: a failure of an X-ray to detect infection does not guarantee that such an infection is not present, but when an infection is indicated on an X-ray it is certainly confirmation of it. With that in mind, the actual number and percentages of infected root canal-treated teeth in the following studies are almost certain to be considerably higher than reported.

Using regular two-dimensional radiographic (X-ray) analysis, researchers in Belgium detected periapical infection in 40.4% of the root canal-treated teeth in 206 patients, while only 6.6% of non-treated teeth showed evidence of infection. Additionally, these researchers reported that 56.7% of the procedures were inadequate.[4] A similar study in Scotland with 319 patients reported periapical infection associated with 50.8% of root canal-treated teeth.[5] Researchers in Turkey reported a root canal treatment failure rate of nearly 68% of the 1,014 teeth examined, based on the detection of periapical infection.[6] And in Germany, an investigation with 323 subjects found periapical infection in 61% of root canal-treated teeth.[7] That same German study reported that, based on the level and density of the root canal fillings, only 14% of the examined root canal-treated teeth were deemed to be adequate according to currently accepted standards.

In addition, a cross-sectional study reported that several other countries had a similarly high incidence of periapical infections as determined by X-ray examination: Denmark at 52%, Lithuania at 44%, Canada at 44% and 51%, Spain at 64.5%, and the United States at 39%.[8]

These studies should alarm patients and professionals alike. Since two-dimensional X-rays often fail to detect periapical infections,

Examination of teeth with "endodontic problems" and "periapical pathology" has shown that just about all root canal-treated teeth, including all of the procedures considered "technically successful," show periapical pathology.

root canal-treated teeth are infected and leak at even higher rates than reported above. At a bare minimum, this is firm evidence of a failure rate substantially higher than claimed by the dental profession.

Additional evidence of infection in root canal-treated teeth is now being revealed by recent developments in 3D cone beam computed tomography X-ray imaging. Using this new technology, examination of teeth with "endodontic problems" and "periapical pathology" has shown that just about all root canal-treated teeth, including all of the procedures considered "technically successful," show periapical pathology (progression of disease) typical for chronic infection of these teeth.

2D X-rays detected infection in 70% of the teeth, the 3D technique discovered infection in 91%.

With conventional two-dimensional dental X-rays, much of this pathology was not visible because the periapical lesions were hidden either in front of or behind the root, or often 2-3 mm away from the radiographic apex of the tooth, thus rendering them undetectable. In one study the 3D technique discovered infection in 21% more root canal-treated teeth than was detected with 2D X-rays. While 2D X-rays detected infection in 70% of the teeth, the 3D technique discovered infection in 91% of the *same* 46 teeth.[9]

Evolving 3D technology serves to show that *the vast majority of root canal-treated teeth have radiological evidence indicating chronic infection*.

This technology is continuing to expand its range of applications and the quality of diagnostic information obtained from it.[10]

Testing for Toxic Teeth

How can we objectively measure the degree of toxicity in root canal-treated teeth? We know that the root canal procedure cannot remove all the bacteria within a tooth and that over time additional bacteria will enter the tooth. So what? The AAE states that any bacteria remaining in the tooth will stay inside the tooth and therefore cannot cause any systemic disease.

Studies have shown that bacteria *do* come out of the root canal-treated tooth into the surrounding periodontal tissues.[11] But more importantly, it is the small molecular weight exotoxins like hydrogen sulfide and methyl thiol that readily migrate out of the root canal-treated tooth. But just how toxic are these exotoxins?

Dr. Boyd Haley developed a test to determine the toxicity of root canal-treated teeth. The process that he developed is called nucleotide photo affinity labeling. He wanted to see if toxins coming out of a root canal-treated tooth would inhibit the activity of five key human enzymes: phosphorylase kinase, phosphorylase A, pyruvate kinase, creatine kinase, and adenylate kinase. The degree of enzyme inhibition would give a representative assessment of the toxicity of this tooth and it's potential systemic impact.

The experimental procedure involved the following:

1) The root portion of an extracted root canal-treated tooth was placed in 1 ml of sterile water and shaken for 1 hour.

2) The tooth was removed and placed in another 1 ml of sterile water and shaken for 1 hour. These two washings would remove anything on the exterior of the root surface.

3) The tooth was then placed in a third 1 ml of sterile water and shaken for 1 hour. This third wash is used to test for enzyme inhibition since any toxins present would have to have come from inside the tooth because the previous two washes removed all external contaminants.

Also, the third wash was used in the toxin assay because the first and second washes always showed extreme levels of toxicity against these five enzymes, and further dilution was required to better comparatively measure their toxicity. The test was designed to both eliminate contaminating toxins from the outside of the tooth, while still showing the clear toxicity from toxins that continue to be eluted from the inside of the tooth in the third wash.

Using the process of nucleotide photo affinity labeling this third wash extract was tested against the five enzymes to determine a level of enzyme inhibition. What Dr. Haley found after studying over 5,000 consecutive extracted root canal-treated teeth was that about 25% of these teeth showed minimal toxicity (less than 5% enzyme inhibition) while others still showed profound tox-

All of the [over 5,000] tested root canal-treated teeth were sufficiently infected to produce toxins.

icity. The primary point to be concluded is that, even with two very prolonged washings before the third washing, measurable toxicity was detected in **100%** of this series of teeth. As toxins in the tooth do **not** naturally occur, this is clear evidence that all of the tested root canal-treated teeth were sufficiently infected to produce toxins.

Dr. Haley also found that albumin was present in this third extract. Albumin is a protein that the body uses in greater amounts in an infected site in an attempt to bind to and neutralize local toxins. So the more albumin that is present in the third wash extract, then generally the higher level of toxicity of that root canal-treated tooth.

Dr. Haley then processed this third wash extract even further to separate the proteins from the small molecular weight toxins. A sample of the third wash extract was processed in a device called a Centricon that uses a filter and a centrifuge to separate out the proteins. This protein-free extract was tested against the same five enzymes used in the first test plus an additional enzyme, acidic fibroblast growth factor. These enzymes were chosen because they all bind ATP, the essential energy molecule in all cells, and they all had different molecular weights so they could be easily separated on gel electrophoresis. Inhibition of these enzymes meant the toxins were directly inhibiting the production of energy and elec-tron donation (antioxidant effect) in the body.

These enzymes were tested against a control of a highly toxic 2 micromolar concentration of hydro-gen sulfide. The tooth extract containing the small molecular weight toxins showed the same level of enzyme inhibition, and therefore the same level of toxicity, as hydrogen sulfide. Some of these toxins could be identified, and others so far have not been identified. Some have a very distinct and offensive odor, and others are odorless.

Dr. Haley also tested samples that were ob-tained from osteonecrotic cavitation surgery and tested these against the same enzymes used in test-ing extracted root canal-treated teeth. He found similar levels of toxicity as well as the presence of metals such as mercury, silver, and cadmium, along with the presence of increased albumin. These cavitations also contained anaerobic bacteria, which released the same toxins that are found in root canal-treated teeth.

Of note, normal teeth extracted for orthodontic purposes never demonstrated any toxicity on Dr. Haley's test.

Dr. Haley has proven that root canal-treated teeth are not healthy. They can release extremely potent exotoxins produced by the bacteria that remain inside the tooth. These toxins:

- ✓ Disseminate throughout the body
- ✓ Do not stay confined inside the tooth as the AAE claims
- ✓ Are deleterious to normal cellular function and
- ✓ Can cause or worsen systemic disease.

Most, If Not All, Root Canal-Treated Teeth Are Infected — Now What?

The official American Association of Endodontists website purports to debunk three common myths concerning root canal treatment. The comment under "Myth #2—Root canal treatment causes illness" provides this comforting verbiage:

"**TRUTH**: There is no valid, scientific evidence
linking root canal-treated teeth and disease elsewhere in the body. A root canal is a safe and effective procedure. When a severe infection in a tooth
requires endodontic treatment, that treatment is
designed to eliminate bacteria from the infected
root canal, prevent reinfection of the tooth and
save the natural tooth."

"The presence of bacteria in teeth and the
mouth has been an accepted fact for many
years. But the presence of bacteria does not
constitute "infection" and is not necessarily a
threat to a person's health. Bacteria are present
in the mouth and teeth at all times, even
in teeth that have never had a cavity or other
trauma. Research shows that *the healthy
immune system takes care of bacteria in a
matter of minutes.*"[12] [emphasis added]

Although the site admits that there are bacteria in the mouth and teeth, it does not admit the
possibility of infection in a root canal-treated tooth.
Plus, it offers a subtle disclaimer by specifying "the
healthy immune system" without really defining
that. But the implication is that the immune system will take care of any residual infection in a root
canal-treated tooth "in a matter of minutes." So if
you are relatively healthy, there's nothing to worry
about, right? Unfortunately, no.

That's the subject of the next chapter...

CHAPTER FOUR

FAULTY FALL-BACK *of Root Canal Treatment*

Can the Immune System Save the Mission?

By now it should be evident that most, if not all, root canal-treated teeth remain infected. Substantiation in the previous chapters confirms that root canal-treated teeth leak bacteria and toxins through both the apical foramen at the tip of the root and the dentinal tubules.[1] And even while endodontists admit that bacteria "might" leak from the treated tooth, they still claim that the procedure is safe and effective, even in the face of this admission.

Here's a quote from the official website of the American Association of Endodontists (AAE):

> "A root canal is a safe and effective procedure. When a severe infection in a tooth requires endodontic treatment, that treatment is designed to eliminate bacteria from the infected root canal, prevent reinfection of the tooth and save

the natural tooth. The presence of bacteria in teeth and the mouth has been an accepted fact for many years. But the presence of bacteria does not constitute 'infection' and is not necessarily a threat to a person's health. Bacteria are present in the mouth and teeth at all times, even in teeth that have never had a cavity or other trauma. Research shows that the healthy immune system takes care of bacteria in a matter of minutes."[2]

This statement essentially concedes that all the bacteria *can't be eliminated from an infected tooth*, and then claims that this reality isn't a health risk because "research shows that the healthy immune system takes care of bacteria in a matter of minutes."

At this point several questions need to be asked:

✓ What does the AAE mean by "take care of"?

✓ Does the immune system "take care of" *all* bacteria? If not, to which bacteria is the AAE referring? What about the clinical cases of brain abscess caused by an infected tooth? Strep throat? Or the long list of other bacterial infections that the immune system should have "taken care" of?

✓ The AAE states that the presence of bacteria does not constitute infection. This is misleading since without a blood supply inside the tooth, a root canal-treated tooth cannot mount an inflammatory response. The lack of an inflammatory response actually allows the bacteria to thrive without the threat of an immune response. Further, although our bodies contain millions of bacteria that do not cause us illness, just like with real estate, it is location, location, location! It is the presence of pathogenic bacteria within tissues that should be normally free of bacteria that causes the problem. How then does the AAE claim that the residual bacteria that caused the need for a root canal in the first place not constitute an infection?

✓ If the immune system "takes care of" all infectious bacteria, why did the tooth become infected in the first place and "require" the root canal procedure? And if the immune system is truly healthy, wouldn't it "take care of" any and all infection in a tooth?

✓ What about the exotoxins created by bacteria, does the immune system "take care of" them, too?

In theory the AAE is depending on effective immune function, which has already failed to prevent or eliminate infection in the tooth. What will enable the immune system to "take care of" this same infection as it is scattered to other parts of the body?

In practice dentists inadvertently admit that the immune system is not able to "take care of" the bacteria released from an infected tooth. These endodontic practitioners frequently and correctly tell a patient that a failure to deal with the infected tooth could eventually have a catastrophic impact on other parts of the body, such as the heart or the brain. (*An untreated, infected tooth can and probably will produce disease in other parts of the body, given enough time. Unfortunately, the root canal treatment cannot effectively eliminate the source of infection.*)

Although toxic shock syndrome can produce dramatic harmful effects at numerous distant sites in the body, the actual focus of toxin production is often hidden.

In the early 20th century, Weston Price, Frank Billings, Ed Rosenow, and others provided copious research that showed a localized infection in a root canal-treated tooth could cause or promote disease in other parts of the body. It is ironic that the very concept that the AAE has tried to discredit has become an argument used to convince a patient of the need for endodontic treatment.

The phenomenon they want to debunk is referred to as "the focal infection theory" which states that a localized infection in the body can initiate and/or promote systemic disease in other parts of the body. Debunking this theory, however, requires the denial of observable facts.

Some bacteria will synthesize and secrete poisons, called exotoxins, in response to oxygen deprivation as well as other environmental changes. Perhaps the most well-known of these exotoxins is produced by the normally innocuous bacteria *Clostridium botulinum.* Every day people all over the world ingest this microorganism on fruits and vegetables without consequence. However, when a small number of these bacteria find their way into a vacuum-packed can and are sealed away from oxygen, the situation changes quickly. Under these conditions the bacteria secrete the deadly botulism exotoxin and taint all the food in the container.

Since it is the exotoxin from the bacteria in this example, and not the bacteria itself that attacks the body, the immune system is less effective in effectively defending itself. The resulting food poisoning can be, and often is, fatal.

Toxic Shock Syndrome: a Deadly Example of a Focal Infection

Toxic shock syndrome is another example of this type of poisoning. This disease was first described in the late 1970's and initially observed in women who used "super absorbent" tampons.

The conditions are ripe for developing toxic shock syndrome when *Staphylococcus aureus* bacteria multiply throughout the absorbent tampon material. In the absence of oxygen these bacteria secrete the TSST-1 exotoxin. The longer the infected tampon is left in place, the higher the likelihood that the toxin will leak out of the tampon and get into the bloodstream. If this happens, the poison can migrate to and damage organs throughout the body.

In *Cecil Textbook of Medicine,* 19th edition, the clinical presentation of toxic shock syndrome is described as follows:

> "The patient, almost always unaware of the focus [origin] of toxin production [the tampon], experiences the abrupt onset of high fever, myalgia [muscle pain], and profuse nausea, vomiting, and watery diarrhea. ...The patient often becomes progressively more ill and is frequently in frank shock when presenting for care. ...Hypotension and frank shock are common and are often associated with acute respiratory distress syndrome [ARDS], acute renal [kidney] failure,

and abnormalities in literally every organ system evaluated."[3]

Why can't the immune system kill these toxin-producing bacteria before they cause disease? The answer is fairly basic. Bacteria gain entrance and grow in the tampon because it is made from a porous substance. They multiply and thrive since fluids can seep in and provide nourishment. But since there is no blood supply in the tampon, these bacteria are protected from the infection-fighting agents of the immune system, such as white blood cells.

These bacteria grow and produce life-threatening exotoxins for which the immune system has little defense. Ultimately, the exotoxins spread to the rest of the body and initiate a toxic shock response in various organs and structures throughout the body.

The actual site of a focal infection can infect and/or poison other parts of the body without exhibiting any symptoms at the originating location.

Toxic shock syndrome is an accelerated model of a focal infection. A bacterial focus at one site in the body subsequently causes disease in one or more distant sites. In the case of toxic shock syndrome, it is the dissemination of the bacterial toxins and not the bacteria themselves that is the primary reason for the development of the disease.

Although toxic shock syndrome can produce dramatic harmful effects at numerous distant sites in the body, the actual focus of toxin production is often hidden. Again referring to *Cecil Textbook of Medicine*, "toxic shock syndrome is almost certainly caused by the production of one or more toxins at the site of a localized and often relatively asymptomatic or unnoticed infection with any strain of *S. aureus* capable of toxin production."[2] In other words, the actual site of a focal infection can infect and/or poison other parts of the body without exhibiting any symptoms at the originating location.

The Immune System Cannot Make the Root Canal Procedure Safe

The comparison between a root canal-treated tooth and a tampon is useful in illustrating the mechanism of initial infection with subsequent dissemination of bacteria and bacterial toxins from that focus of infection. It highlights the devastating consequences of providing a microorganism-friendly environment that is sequestered from the immune system. It also demonstrates how a root canal-treated tooth can actually be highly toxic and yet remain "asymptomatic."

A root canal procedure is almost always performed when the normally sterile pulp canal becomes infected with bacteria and then becomes painful. These bacteria invade the pulp and migrate down the root canal space and into the porous tooth structure composed of countless dentinal tubules. There, just like with a tampon, the bacteria continue to grow in the warm, moist, dark, and now bacteria-friendly environment. Moreover, once the pulp tissue becomes necrotic, the bacteria infecting the tooth are now effectively out of reach of the body's immune system. Antibiotics are also of little help since there is no blood supply to effectively deliver them to the infection.

> *Just like with a tampon... the bacteria infecting the tooth are now effectively out of reach of the body's immune system.*

Newer tampon designs, as well as changing them frequently, can significantly reduce the risk of developing toxic shock syndrome associated with tampons. The problem with a root canal-treated tooth is that it is an integral part of your body and cannot be changed. The infected tooth is a permanent focus of infection that has the potential to cause disease throughout the body for as long as it remains.

The predominant *Streptococci* bacteria in infected teeth are not the same strain seen in toxic shock syndrome. But when deprived of oxygen, as is the case in the root canal-treated tooth, they frequently produce very potent toxins that can cause a low-grade, continuous type of toxic shock. Such a situation can eventually manifest as any of a multitude of different diseases, depending upon the genetic predispositions or "weaknesses" of the affected patients.

It is unlikely that proponents of endodontic treatment will accept the logic in this comparison of a root canal-treated tooth with the toxic shock syndrome. The AAE website claims that there is no scientific evidence that root canal-treated teeth actually cause disease. Contrary to the AAE claim, however, there is plenty of scientific evidence that root canal-treated teeth cause disease. That is the subject of the next chapter.

CHAPTER FIVE

IMPACT *of Root Canal Treatment*

Disease Connection Confirmed

INTRODUCTION

A statement like the one that still appears on the official American Association of Endodontists (AAE) website, even as this book goes to print, is quite disturbing for a couple of reasons. It reads,

> **TRUTH**: There is no valid, scientific evidence linking root canal-treated teeth and disease elsewhere in the body. A root canal is a safe and effective procedure.[1]

At first glance, this categorical statement seems to settle the issue once and for all: the root canal procedure is safe and effective. Period.

However, contrary to the AAE's claim of "no valid, scientific evidence," there is a significant and growing body of compelling evidence linking root canal-treated teeth to systemic disease. Much of this research has been published in peer-reviewed ***dental*** journals.

Either the AAE is ignorant of relevant and valid research occurring on its own turf—a thought that should trouble its members—or it chooses to reject the evidence because acceptance would invalidate previous claims by the AAE that root canal-treated teeth pose no possible systemic health risks.

"Innocent until proven guilty" does not apply in matters of health and safety.

But even if the research did fail to demonstrate a link between root canal-treated teeth and systemic diseases, "innocent until proven guilty" does not apply in matters of health and safety. To leap from "there's no evidence of danger" to "therefore it's safe" is deceptive. At present there's "no valid, scientific evidence" linking roller-skating down an interstate during rush hour with death or injury, but that certainly doesn't mean that such an activity is safe or advisable.

This chapter will present and discuss a few of a large number of valid scientific studies that *do* link root canal-treated teeth to disease—links to heart disease, stroke, dementia, diabetes, lung disease, kidney disease, cancer, and other conditions.

THE HISTORICAL AND SCIENTIFIC CONTEXT

Links between oral infections and disease were first identified in the early 1900's. At that time, a host of medical researchers, including Charles Mayo (founder of the Mayo Clinic), Frank Billings,

Weston Price, Ed Rosenow, and several others were independently seeing an unmistakable link between systemic disease and various strains of bacteria. Notably, a vast majority of these pathogens seemed to originate from oral sources in and around infected teeth.

Diligent work by all of these researchers pointed to the same conclusion: many degenerative diseases can be initiated by specific pathogens. Each pathogen seemed to have an affinity to a particular organ or structure in the body. Meticulous bacteriological work by over thirty different researchers reported the same correlations. At the same time it was noted that the anaerobic (non-oxygen-containing) environment inside root canal-treated teeth was particularly instrumental in the development and spread of these virulent strains of bacteria that would initiate seemingly unrelated degenerative diseases in particular tissues and organs in the body.

Charles Mayo (founder of the Mayo Clinic), Frank Billings, Weston Price, Ed Rosenow, and several others were independently seeing an unmistakable link between systemic disease and various strains of bacteria.

As pulpless (root canal-treated) teeth were extracted from patients with a variety of systemic diseases, cultures were made from the bacteria obtained from the inside of these teeth and then injected into laboratory animals (usually rabbits). With very few exceptions, the rabbits would quickly develop the same disease as the patient from whom the tooth was extracted. Thousands of experiments were performed in a variety of ways by many different researchers, and all were finding very similar results.

These toxins [from root canal-treated teeth], when isolated and injected into laboratory animals, were consistently lethal.

In addition, studies were conducted using extracted root canal-treated teeth that were ground and scrubbed to remove all bacteria, leaving only the toxins these bacteria had produced. These toxins, when isolated and injected into laboratory animals, were consistently lethal.

In the same way, samples from healthy extracted teeth that had been surrounded by healthy periodontal tissues were cultured. These samples produced few bacterial colonies, and when bacteria did grow, they never demonstrated the virulence found in cultures taken from pulpless teeth. The negative implications of these observations provided a serious indictment against root canal treatments. In fact, these pathological findings were so compelling that in 1913 Dr. Mayo issued this challenge to dentists:

> It falls upon the dentist and oral surgeon to study the diseased conditions of the mouth. The work is

discouraging, but it must be kept up, as eventually it will have its effect. The next great leap in medical progress in the line of preventive medicine should be made by the dentists. The question is will they do it?[2]

They did not. They quickly covered their eyes and ears. Refusing to see or hear any evidence that threatened their dental practices, they only looked for ways to silence the critics.

A Fraud Provides Cover for Dental Industry

In the late 1930s, defenders of the root canal procedure were desperately looking for a way to refute the mounting evidence against root canal treatments. Their need just happened to converge with the professional jealousy of a doctor named W. L. Holman. His envy of Ed Rosenow's acclaim energized an obsession with discrediting Rosenow's work. Much like certain cancers tend to metastasize to specific organs, Rosenow's research clearly demonstrated that certain bacteria show an affinity for invading specific bodily tissues.

For example, Rosenow took bacteria from patients with stomach ulcers and injected these bacteria isolates into laboratory animals. Sixty percent of these laboratory animals developed stomach ulcers as compared to only 17% that developed stomach ulcers when injected with bacteria isolated from patients with various other diseases. Repeated experiments by Rosenow and others with over 10,000 laboratory animals showed the same findings of specific bacteria affecting specific tissues, which came to be known as **elective localization**.

Holman, however, performed no bacteriological research himself. He did not question or analyze the research methods used by Rosenow, nor did he put forward any argument against the validity of the collected data. He simply reorganized all the data to suit his purposes. Then he recalculated results to completely obscure the obvious statistical correlation between **specific** diseases and **particular** pathogens.

> Holman's statistical sleight of hand **never** claimed that infections in root canal-treated teeth were not responsible for causing disease in other parts of the body.

Holman's statistical sleight of hand **never** claimed that infections in root canal-treated teeth were not responsible for causing disease in other parts of the body. And although completely invalid, his dishonest dismissal of Rosenow's meticulous work in particular provided the ammunition that worried dentists needed to discredit any connection between the root canal procedure and systemic disease risk. This disheartening story is well-documented in S. Hale Shakman's dissertation, *Medicine's Grandest Fraud*.[3]

For decades modern dentistry has relied on the work of Holman and those who followed him, using conclusions based on flawed calculations, to persuade dentists, dental students, and the public that the root canal procedure is safe. However, new research is now confirming the same disease links that were first reported by Rosenow, Price, and others.

The Meticulous Research of Weston Price

Weston Price was a dentist who performed many experiments that very clearly demonstrated that both bacteria and their associated toxins readily escape from a root canal-treated tooth. In several of his experiments, he surgically implanted extracted root canal-treated teeth under the skin of rabbits. These teeth were always highly toxic. He found that if the rabbits did not quickly die from the overwhelming toxicity of the implanted teeth, they typically developed the same diseases that plagued the humans from whom the teeth had been extracted. He repeated these experiments over and over and continued to obtain the same results.

If the rabbits did not quickly die from... implanted [root canal-treated] teeth, they typically developed the same diseases that plagued the humans from whom the teeth had been extracted.

Price would repeatedly verify not only the enormous toxicity of these extracted root canal-treated teeth, he also demonstrated that there existed an uncanny specificity of these teeth to reproduce the different diseases of their human donors in their rabbit recipients.

For example, if a patient presented with a kidney infection that resolved after extraction of a root canal-treated tooth, and this tooth was implanted under the skin of a rabbit, the rabbit would develop the same kidney infection. Dr. Price found that various bacteria had an affinity for specific body tissues and would tend to migrate there. This is the phenomenon called elective localization, a term coined by its discoverer, Dr. Edward Rosenow, as noted earlier.

As further proof that it was the infection in extracted root canal-treated teeth that was responsible for the development of systemic disease, he also implanted **uninfected** extracted teeth under the skin or muscle of rabbits. He also implanted sterilized objects such as coins to see if just the presence of a foreign body might cause disease. In all such implants nothing of consequence happened to these laboratory animals. The implanted objects, either uninfected teeth or other foreign bodies, eventually became encapsulated in a cyst-like sack and remained sterile. All of the rabbits remained healthy.

Price also reported numerous dramatic improvements in cases of systemic disease following the removal of root canal-treated teeth. Unfortunately, the failure of other researchers to observe similar improvements is frequently used in the attempt to discredit all his research.

For example, researchers came to the conclusion that no benefit accrued to 47 out of 52 patients with rheumatoid arthritis after the infected teeth were removed.[4] This study is cited to disprove the link between root canal-treated teeth and systemic disease. The secondary infection involved in the rheumatoid arthritis likely had already been seeded and established at the time of tooth extraction. Ongoing antigen-antibody inflammatory reactions, along with the chronic physical changes of the disease, can continue to feed the inflammatory response even after the initiating infection is resolved. This is called molecular mimicry. If the invading bacteria share at least one antigen-presenting protein with a similar protein in the normal body tissue, the immune system can continue to attack that body tissue after the initial infection has resolved. None of these extracted teeth were implanted into rabbits, so the experimental model of Dr. Price was never invalidated.

The fallacy of this argument becomes clear upon closer examination. The observation that the arthritis fails to resolve after the removal of a root canal-treated tooth does not settle the question of whether the infection in the teeth was in any way responsible for that arthritis. Most systemic diseases, once established with other resulting physical and chemical abnormalities, are not resolved by the removal of the initiating factor(s). The study only really proved that rheumatoid arthritis is a multifactorial disease in many individuals, and that it is unlikely that any intervention will ever reverse the chronic physical deformities and much of the symptomatology that accompany such a disease.

Exotoxins produced by the infecting bacteria are the main cause of pathogenicity in root canal-treated teeth.

For example, when high blood pressure results in kidney disease, suddenly bringing the hypertension under control does not automatically undo the damage to the kidney. In like manner, just because a chronic, 30-year cigarette smoker stops smoking upon a diagnosis of lung cancer, doesn't mean that the cancer will resolve. Nor does the fact that his cancer remains in any way exonerate cigarette smoke from any role in the development of that cancer.

Price also provided confirmation for another reality: Exotoxins produced by the infecting bacteria are the main cause of pathogenicity in root canal-treated teeth. To demonstrate this he made extracts from ground-up root canal-treated teeth. All the bacteria were filtered out, leaving just the soluble extract. When this bacteria-free extract was injected into rabbits, they would often get sick or die sooner than when they were exposed to the skin implantation of the entire tooth that still contained live bacteria.

Root Canal-Treated Teeth: Hotbeds of Pathogens and Toxins

The overall number and diversity of microorganisms found in dental pulp infections and root canal-treated teeth is staggering. Over 460 different bacteria have been identified in these teeth,[5,6] with a high preponderance of anaerobic species.[7] Among these bacteria are even included a wide array of spirochetes of the genus *Treponema*.[8]

The AAE states that any bacteria remaining in a root canal-treated tooth will remain inside the tooth and can never travel to other sites in the body. Contrary to this claim, however, research presented elsewhere in this book and in this chapter shows that these bacteria almost never remain sequestered inside the root canal-treated tooth. Irrefutable DNA evidence, presented below, shows that these dental pathogens, present both in root canal-treated teeth as well as in the infections around such teeth, commonly travel to and embed in various bodily tissues.

> *DNA evidence... shows that these dental pathogens... in root canal-treated teeth... commonly travel to and embed in various bodily tissues.*

But more importantly, these bacteria can produce extremely potent exotoxins that easily migrate out of the root canal-treated tooth and disseminate throughout the body.

Bacterial Toxins Produced in the Root Canal-Treated Tooth

By definition, pathogenic bacteria traveling throughout the body present a serious health risk, but that systemic danger is increased further by the toxins that these pathogens produce. Researchers divide these poisonous substances into two types: endotoxins and exotoxins.

Endotoxins are large molecules comprised of repeating carbohydrate chains attached to a lipid. They are found on the outer membranes of gram-negative bacteria and produce a strong immune response in animals. Generally, endotoxins are only released when the bacteria die. They can cause disease but they are rarely fatal.

Two recent investigations found them [endotoxins] in 100% of such [infected] teeth examined.

The majority of research on the pathogenicity of root canal-treated teeth has focused on endotoxins because they are easier to study than exotoxins. Endotoxins have been documented to always be present in the infected pulp tissue of teeth that have not received root canal treatments. Two recent investigations found them in 100% of such teeth examined. One study found endotoxins in 21 of 21 infected pulp tissues, and the other study found them in 30 of 30 infected pulp tissues.[9,10]

Exotoxins are created inside living bacteria and generally secreted, although they can also be released upon death of the bacteria. These toxins can destroy cells and disrupt cellular metabolism throughout the body. Well-known examples of exotoxins include botulinum toxin that causes botulism, diphtheria toxin capable of causing myocarditis, and tetanospasmin toxin that produces tetanus. Exotoxins are usually much more toxic than endotoxins and can readily cause cell death and even death of the host animal or patient. Exotoxins can act on the enzymes inside a cell while endotoxins cannot.

Endotoxins are present in a root canal-treated tooth, and now work by Dr. Boyd Haley has demonstrated that exotoxins are present as well.

Research cited above shows that endotoxins are present in a root canal-treated tooth, and now work by Dr. Boyd Haley has demonstrated that exotoxins are present as well (see Chapter Three). Since a root canal-treated tooth cannot be sterilized, the exotoxin-producing bacteria present in an infected tooth before root canal treatment will remain in the tooth after the procedure.

Post-extraction examination shows that all root canal-treated teeth can function as a protected reservoir of anaerobic bacteria, endotoxins, and exotoxins. These pathogenic bacteria, and, especially the small molecule exotoxins, readily migrate out of the root canal-treated tooth. The idea that such a pool of pathogens and toxins poses no systemic risk defies reason.

THE PATHOGENIC EQUIVALENCY BETWEEN PERIODONTITIS AND ROOT CANAL-TREATED TEETH

Periodontitis: "Smoking Gun" Evidence Linking Root Canal-Treated Teeth to Systemic Disease

An infection in the gum tissue that also involves the jawbone is called periodontitis. When the periodontal infection reaches the apex (tip) of the tooth's root, it becomes a more serious infection that is called apical periodontitis.

General periodontitis develops as bacteria around a tooth invade and proliferate in the space between the tooth and the gum (the sulcus). These bacteria release enzymes that cause direct tissue damage as they effectively "unzip" the fibers attaching the gum tissue to both the tooth and the jawbone. When these migrating bacteria infect the jawbone and cause it to resorb (dissolve), the damage becomes visible on an X-ray and the condition is diagnosed as periodontitis.

The bacteria continue to release enzymes and toxins while they migrate further down the sulcus. During this migration, more and more of the jawbone surrounding the tooth is resorbed. These colonies of bacteria become more anaerobic as they go deeper in the tissues where the oxygen concentration is low.

All root canal-treated teeth can function as a protected reservoir of infectious anaerobic bacteria, endotoxins, and exotoxins.

Apical periodontitis can develop in two different ways. The first way occurs when a periodontal infection, as just described, is left untreated. Over time the infection can progress to the root tip of the tooth as bacterial enzymes continue to dissolve the bone surrounding the tooth root. Apical periodontitis can also develop when an infection in the pulp of the tooth or in the dentinal tubules of a root canal-treated tooth escapes through the apical foramen.

Apical periodontitis appears as a dark area on an X-ray due to the bone resorption caused by the infection. When the infection originates from inside the tooth, it will usually be confined to the area around the tip of the tooth. In the case of apical periodontitis caused by advanced periodontal disease, the dark area of infection seen on X-ray will extend from the tip of the root completely up the side of the tooth root.

Except for the rare case of aseptic apical periodontitis caused by traumatic injury, apical periodontitis **always** involves infection of the tooth pulp, even if the tooth was initially healthy.[11] This is because once the bacteria migrate down the root to the area surrounding the root's tip they now have easy access into the tooth through the apical foramen.

Bacteria can also gain entrance into the tooth directly through the exterior of the root surface. Even before a periodontal infection reaches the apical foramen, bacteria found in the infected periodontal tissues surrounding a tooth root can migrate into the tooth root's dentinal tubules directly through the cementum that encases the root portion of the tooth. At this point the bacteria are free to invade the dentinal tubules and may proliferate within the tooth and cause the tooth to die.

3D X-rays have found that up to 91% of root canal-treated teeth are still infected.

A root and pulp infection that precipitates apical periodontitis is responsible for much of the pain that sends someone to the endodontist in the first place, and then it becomes the reason for performing a root canal procedure. Foundationally, a diagnosis of "apical periodontitis" really means that the tooth is **already infected**. Unfortunately, as discussed in Chapters Two and Three, the root canal procedure never clears up the infection, although it will usually relieve the associated pain. In addition, some of the same bacteria that caused the initial infection can always be expected to remain in the surrounding bone even after the root canal procedure is performed, in spite of a normal, or less abnormal, X-ray appearance.

Any study that looks at the negative clinical impact of periodontitis... parallels the toxic and pathogenic realities of a root canal-treated tooth.

Many of the studies regarding the low success rate of root canal-treated teeth discussed in Chapter Three cited the presence of apical periodontitis under a root canal-treated tooth as **confirmation** that root canal treatment had **failed** to eliminate the infection.[12] And although X-rays are unable to detect all such failures, 3D X-rays have found that up to 91% of root canal-treated teeth demonstrate pathology indicative of infection.[13]

Since a vast majority of root canal-treated teeth have been associated with periodontitis, any study that looks at the negative clinical impact of periodontitis—**at the very minimum**—parallels the toxic and pathogenic realities of a root canal-treated tooth. Most likely the impact of a root canal-treated tooth is much worse.

Any persistence of periodontitis remaining after a root canal is performed, which would be best detected with 3D X-ray, will continue to have *similar toxicity* and negative clinical impact as if the infected tooth were left untreated. The only difference is that the amount of infected material will be reduced in volume immediately after a root canal procedure.

What's the difference between the accepted health risks from the pathogens and toxins found in periodontitis and those of a root canal-treated tooth?

However, this benefit will be offset over time by the increased toxicity of the root canal-treated tooth due to the alteration of the bacteria in the anaerobic environment within the dentinal tubules and the inevitable proliferation of the pathogens. In addition, over time, more and more bacteria will migrate into the tooth, increasing the bacterial concentration even further without the normal fluid flow within the dentinal tubules to keep these bacteria out.[14]

And, not surprisingly, bacteria that migrate in also migrate out. This is also true of the small molecule exotoxins produced within the root canal-treated tooth. They can easily migrate through the cementum as well as through the tooth apex.

While the AAE states that there is no valid evidence linking root canal-treated teeth to systemic disease, dentists generally acknowledge the scores of studies that demonstrate periodontitis-systemic disease links. *What's the difference between the accepted health risks from the pathogens and toxins found in periodontitis and those of a root canal-treated tooth?* Only this: the bacteria and toxins in a root canal-treated tooth tend to be much more virulent and dangerous, and they are more readily delivered into the body by chewing.

This pathological equivalency means that all the diseases researchers have linked to periodontitis can logically be ascribed to infected tooth canal-treated teeth.

For decades the dental industry has acknowledged the health risks associated with periodontitis. In fact, the bacteria associated with these health risks prompt many dentists to prescribe antibiotics to some of their patients prior to treatment. And the same infectious bacteria that cause periodontitis are nearly always present in a root canal-treated tooth.

Whether a particular pathogen colonizes in the jawbone and gum tissues surrounding a tooth or inside a root canal-treated tooth, this microbe is pathologically equivalent wherever it ends up and therefore presents the same systemic risks.

This pathological equivalency means that all the diseases researchers have linked to

periodontitis can logically be ascribed to infected root canal-treated teeth.

Anyone who resists this conclusion needs to answer the following questions:

- ✓ Aren't the same pathogens that caused the initial periodontal infection responsible for any infection that remains after the root canal procedure is performed?
- ✓ Why would a periodontal infection that has been linked with systemic disease prior to treatment suddenly be released from that association if the infection remains in or around the tooth after the root canal treatment?

Dentists readily discuss the coronary heart disease risks associated with periodontal infection and aggressively treat it. At the same time they persist in performing—and defending as "safe"—a procedure that allows the same infection to remain in a root canal-treated tooth that has been effectively disconnected from the body's infection detection and healing systems. And the root canal-treated tooth is capable of continuously delivering the associated pathogens and toxins to the body.

"A growing body of scientific evidence has shown that severe periodontitis may enhance susceptibility to certain important systemic diseases..."

RECENT SCIENTIFIC EVIDENCE LINKING ROOT CANAL-TREATED TEETH TO SYSTEMIC DISEASE

Modern Science Recognizes the Link Between Periodontitis and Systemic Diseases

For decades the dental industry has tried to discredit any association between root canal treatment and systemic disease. Many of their efforts have focused on attempting to discredit Dr. Weston Price. He has been a primary target because his work meticulously demonstrated a relationship between infected teeth—both untreated and root canal-treated—and systemic diseases. The AAE website makes this telling statement:

> **But what about Dr. Price?** This is a good example of how the Internet can give new life to long-dispelled theories. Believe it or not, the misinformation about root canals that is found on the Internet is still based on Dr. Price's century-old, discredited research.[15]

The AAE would like everyone to believe that the Internet is responsible for resurrecting the "long-dispelled" theory that links infected teeth and infected root canal-treated teeth with systemic disease. Could it be that the theory won't die because "modern scientific research" is discovering the same connections identified by Price in the first place? A study of the medical and dental literature by independent researchers demonstrates that the relationship is very real, so real that a new specialty called Periodontal Medicine is emerging. Here are a few quotes from the medical literature showing this very reality:

> A growing body of scientific evidence has shown that severe periodontitis may enhance susceptibility to certain important systemic diseases and conditions, for example, cardiovascular disease, diabetes mellitus, adverse pregnancy outcomes, and pulmonary infections. The clinical implications of the emerging specialty of **periodontal medicine** for dental and medical practitioners are postulated.[16] [emphasis added]

"Recent studies have indicated that periodontitis may have an unfathomed effect on the systemic health."

Periodontitis has been attributed to produce a low-grade systemic inflammatory condition. The link of periodontitis to various systemic disorders has led to the evolution of a new branch termed as "**periodontal medicine.**"[17] [emphasis added]

Recent studies have indicated that periodontitis may have an unfathomed effect on the systemic health. A vivid exploration of the cryptic mechanisms linking periodontitis to systemic disorders has ensued into the development of a new branch termed "**periodontal medicine.**"[18] [emphasis added]

It is not a coincidence that modern scientific research is now discovering that cardiovascular disease, pulmonary infections, rheumatoid arthritis, and other systemic diseases are linked to periodontal disease. This old correlation will not die, not because the Internet keeps it alive, but because it is ***true***.

Periodontitis (and Therefore Root Canal-Treated Teeth) Linked to Coronary Heart Disease

Solid research in the last few years substantiates the periodontitis—heart disease link.[19,20,21,22,23,24,25] One investigator's systematic review of the research regarding the relationship between periodontitis and cardiovascular disease echoes a common theme in the dental and medical literature:

> Efforts to test causality in the relationship between periodontitis and CVD [cardiovascular disease] are ongoing. Evidence to date is consistent with the notion that severe generalized periodontitis causes systemic inflammation and endothelial dysfunction. Periodontitis has effects that go beyond the oral cavity and its treatment and prevention may contribute to the prevention of atherosclerosis.[26]

"Periodontitis has effects that go beyond the oral cavity and its treatment and prevention may contribute to the prevention of atherosclerosis."

Interestingly, Weston Price warned of the close connection between infected teeth and diseases of the heart in 1923. In one of many cases that he treated, he reported about a 15-year-old boy with endocarditis. Endocarditis is an infection that typically affects heart valves. Initially, this boy complained of a severe toothache in a first molar. The tooth was extracted and pulp cultures were taken. Cultures identified the bacteria as a streptococcus, and then some of the cultured organisms were injected into 30 rabbits. In a matter of a few days, twenty-eight (93%) of the rabbits developed endocarditis and died. Acute endocarditis claimed the boy's life about seven months later.[27]

This infection was found in a pulp-infected tooth that did not have a root canal treatment. Although this tooth had not undergone root canal treatment, the same type of organisms can be assumed to remain in the dentinal tubules and lateral canals after a root canal procedure is performed. Price reported on other similar cases with infected teeth, some root canal-treated and others not, and their observed link to heart diseases.

Another individual, a 49-year-old man who was experiencing pain in his chest, was diagnosed as having myocarditis (inflammation of the heart). This patient was found to have two infected molars. Anaerobic cultures made from these teeth were injected into two rabbits. One rabbit died in twelve hours and the second rabbit's heart became large and flabby. A large, flabby heart is often the result of a rapidly progressive myocarditis. Upon removal of these infected teeth all of this patient's symptoms improved.[28]

Infective endocarditis is the most definitive and well-documented example of focal infection, and both aerobic and anaerobic bacteria have caused it. Many patients who have experienced infective endocarditis had no prior knowledge of heart valve damage, which is often a predisposing factor in acquiring this infection.

In the 1950s, the American Dental Association summarily dismissed Price's research. Decades later, researchers are again reporting the connection between infected teeth and diseases of the heart.

Decades later, [after the ADA summarily dismissed Price's research] researchers are again reporting the connection between infected teeth and diseases of the heart.

Many heart surgeons today include an oral examination before operating. Since virtually all root canal-treated teeth are infected (see Chapter Three), this presents a serious health risk for all those who are already at risk for heart disease.

The bacteria commonly found in the mouth can cause an aggregation (clumping) of platelets, which can also contribute to the blocking of an artery that can result in heart attack or stroke. *In vitro* studies have demonstrated that two bacteria species found around the teeth, *Streptococcus sanguis* and *Porphyromonas gingivalis*, can cause the clotting of blood associated with heart attack. At the same time, animal studies showed that the presence of these bacteria resulted in dramatic changes in blood pressure, respiratory rate, and heartbeat within 30 minutes of injection into the bloodstream.[29]

> *Streptococcus sanguis, which are found in infected teeth including root canal-treated teeth, contribute to endocarditis as well as to the formation of blood clots.*

An *in vivo* study sought to evaluate the role of periodontal infection and bacterial burden as it relates to the development of acute coronary syndrome. The periodontal species investigated included *Streptococcus intermedius, Streptococcus sanguis, Streptococcus anginosus, Tannerella forsythia, Treponema denticola*, and *Porphyromonas gingivalis*. Since a significantly higher oral bacterial load was observed in patients with acute coronary syndrome versus patients without it, the researchers concluded that the oral bacterial load is a possible risk factor in the development of this disease.[30]

Earlier research demonstrated that *Streptococcus sanguis*, which are found in infected teeth including root canal-treated teeth, contribute to endocarditis as well as to the formation of blood clots. The investigators concluded that the results "explain the additional contributed risk of periodontitis to MI [myocardial infarction, or heart attack]."[31]

Research has also found a **large majority** of human plaque samples taken from the carotid artery contain organisms from dental infections. The investigators concluded "periodontal pathogens are present in atherosclerotic plaques where, like other infectious microorganisms such as *C. pneumoniae*, may play a role in the development and progression of atherosclerosis leading to coronary vascular disease."[32]

An investigation looking at the interrelationship between medical and dental health found that individuals with dental disease have a high prevalence of coronary heart disease.[33] Other researchers found the same heart disease correlation in a 14-year follow-up of 9,760 individuals with periodontitis.[34]

Patients with chronic apical periodontitis had a 2.79 times higher risk of developing coronary artery disease.

Researchers have now independently correlated apical periodontitis with coronary heart disease. These investigators found that patients with chronic apical periodontitis had a *2.79 times higher* risk of developing coronary artery disease.[35]

In a study specifically called "Dental Atherosclerosis Risk in Communities" investigators found
that periodontitis is a risk factor for atherosclerosis and its clinical manifestations, including plaque
buildup in the carotid arteries.[36] Another investigation into the relationship between periodontal disease and coronary heart disease found the subjects
with known infections around the teeth were over
30% more likely to have coronary heart disease
after correcting for all other risk factors such as
smoking and obesity.[37]

The link between periodontitis and coronary
heart disease is well-documented and has been
widely accepted for years. Now research is independently confirming the same heart disease link to chronic apical periodontitis.[38] In 2006 investigators found that
X-ray evidence of infection in the pulps of root canal-treated teeth was associated with the more rapid appearance of
coronary heart disease.[39] A more recent study examined
the dental status of individuals who had already experienced a
myocardial infarction, finding more "inflammatory
processes" of "endodontic origin" in this group versus what was found in a healthy control group.[40] In
the *Journal of Endodontics,* a subspecialty dentistry

*X-ray evidence of
infection in the pulps
of root canal-treated
teeth was associated
with the more
rapid appearance
of coronary heart
disease.*

journal dedicated to root canal treatment research, the researchers found that individuals who presented with "lesions of endodontic origin" or just "pulpal inflammation" had an increased risk of coronary heart disease.[41]

A substantial body of research now exists that further documents the direct link between dental pathogens and atherosclerotic plaques that lead to heart attack. Researchers have consistently found a wide variety of pathogens and microorganisms in the atherosclerotic lesions in patients with chronic coronary artery disease. Bacterial DNA was found in the atherectomy specimens of **100%** of 38 patients with coronary disease. Over **50 different species** of bacteria contributed to this DNA presence, and individual plaques typically had between 10 and 15 **different** bacterial DNAs.[42] In 35 of 38 atherosclerosis patients fungal DNA was found, with each patient typically having from 2 to 9 different fungal species.[43]

> *Researchers have consistently found a wide variety of [dental] pathogens and microorganisms in the atherosclerotic lesions in patients with chronic coronary artery disease.*

Without the awareness that all root canal-treated teeth are infected, researchers have asserted that bacterial DNA "typical for endodontic infection" was present in over 75% of the blood clots aspirated from acutely blocked coronary arteries in patients with acute myocardial infarction. Furthermore, the bacterial DNA content in the clots was *16-fold higher* than that found in blood samples collected, likely indicating the direct "seeding" of the blood clot from the chronically infected/inflamed endothelial wall and underlying plaque, as documented in the studies above.[44]

77% of [atherosclerotic plaques from patients with chronic periodontitis]... contained periodontitis-associated bacteria.

An investigation with chronic periodontitis patients showed that in those with atherosclerotic plaques, 77% of those plaques contained periodontitis-associated bacteria. The researchers also noted "the presence of an active inflammatory process expressed by a significantly higher bleeding index in those patients in whom the examined bacterial species were found in atherosclerotic plaque."[45]

Considerable evidence suggests that bacteria from periodontal infections, as well as their toxic byproducts, induce systemic inflammation leading to the development of cardiovascular disease.[46] This inflammation causes damage to the endothelial lining of the blood vessel walls. The growth of these bacteria and associated toxin-induced damage likely cause an increase in the release of inflammatory mediators known as cytokines. Cytokines can help promote atherosclerosis, the disease process that gradually narrows and eventually blocks off blood flow in arteries. In addition to possibly initiating the inflammation in arterial walls, research also suggests that periodontal bacteria may also enhance and **maintain** that inflammation.[47]

Ironically, the very publication (*Journal of the American Dental Association*) that claims to have "debunked" any and all relationship between root canal treatment and disease has recently published a study with a very different conclusion. In this study the 6,651 participants were asked if they knew whether any of their teeth had received root canal treatments. The entire group was also screened for a history of clearly established coronary heart disease (CHD).

Simply having had a root canal procedure done significantly increases the chances of coronary heart disease.

The conclusion of the study was that participants "...with a greater self-reported history of ET (endodontically-treated teeth, also known as root canal-treated teeth) were more likely to have CHD than were those reporting no history of ET." Furthermore, this conclusion was corrected for the other major risk factors such as smoking, obesity, and high blood pressure.[48] At least two other groups of investigators have reported similar findings.[49,50]

The above three studies are especially significant because they make a direct connection between just **having** root canal-treated teeth present in the mouth with having a clear and significantly increased chance of heart attack. There is no mention in these studies that the root canals need to be "infected," "failed," "symptomatic," "inflamed," or "associated with incident lesions" on X-ray. Instead, these studies simply make the powerful point that, regardless of how technically "successful" the procedure was, **_simply having had a root canal procedure done significantly increases the chances of coronary heart disease._**

Periodontitis (and Therefore Root Canal-Treated Teeth) Linked to Strokes and Other Cardiovascular Health Risks

Stroke patients with advanced periodontitis had greater neurological impairment at the time of admission to the hospital as well as worse outcomes at the time of hospital discharge.

It is generally accepted that high blood pressure (hypertension) is a risk factor associated with kidney diseases as well as heart disease, stroke, embolisms, and aneurysms. A review of several cross-sectional studies demonstrated a clear link between high blood pressure and periodontitis.[51] Other studies link periodontitis to increased mass in the left ventricle (left ventricular hypertrophy) as well as to hypertension.[52,53] Weston Price also reported and demonstrated this periodontitis-hypertension link in 1923 as well as its link to endocarditis, angina pectoris, heart block, myocarditis, and other heart conditions.[54]

Ischemic stroke is a damaging brain event caused by a restriction of blood supply. Periodontitis is universally considered an independent risk factor for this type of event.[55] Researchers reported that stroke patients with advanced periodontitis had greater neurological impairment at the time of admission to the hospital as well as worse outcomes at the time of hospital discharge.[56]

Men under the age of 65 with a history of apical periodontitis have a greater risk of having a stroke.

Men under the age of 65 with a history of apical periodontitis have a greater risk of having a stroke. That was the conclusion of researchers who reviewed X-ray records of 1,137 veteran men who had been followed by dentists at the VA for an average of 34 years.[57] A similar study with periodontal disease patients concluded, "the present results indicate that periodontal disease is associated with the development of early atherosclerotic carotid lesions."[58]

Periodontal bacteremia is the presence of bacteria from periodontal infection that enter the blood. A study of a large medical and dental database in

Tokyo reported that periodontal bacteremia "may play an important role in the development of various vascular diseases, such as Buerger's disease, atherosclerosis and varicose veins."[59]

The bacteria associated with chronic periodontitis strongly promote atherosclerosis, stroke, and heart attack.

Research also shows that a "wide variety of bacteria, including oral bacteria, was found to colonize aortic aneurysms and may play a role in their development."[60]

In another study, two groups of patients, one with chronic periodontitis and the other with no history of tooth infection were compared for cardiovascular health risk factors in the blood. The researchers found that those with chronic periodontitis had increased serum cholesterol and LDL levels.[61] The association of periodontitis with increased serum cholesterol, as well as increased triglyceride levels, has been reported by many others.[62,63,64,65]

The bacteria associated with chronic periodontitis strongly promote atherosclerosis, stroke, and heart attack through a series of mechanisms. These bacteria produce toxins that break down tissues and cause the release of acute phase proteins from the liver like fibrinogen and C-reactive protein. When tissues break down and start dying, the body initiates an inflammatory response in an effort to repair the damaged tissue.

When the bacteria and toxin presence is high and contained in a small vascular area, the inflammatory response and release of acute phase proteins lead to attempted repair of the tissue, which can then promote initiation of atherosclerotic changes if not self-limited. However, when the bacteria and toxin presence is ongoing, as with chronic periodontitis, the continued inflammation makes the developed plaque grow and eventually become unstable. In this state, the plaque is prone to breaking off and causing a heart attack or stroke. It is not always the most occluded arteries that cause the heart attack but rather the "hot" inflamed unstable plaques that are the most dangerous. The potentially lethal impact of this condition is further enhanced by the increased platelet clumping and blood clotting that these periodontal bacteria initiate.

Individuals with periodontitis were 2.8 times as likely to develop pneumonia in the hospital.

Periodontitis (and Therefore Root Canal-Treated Teeth) Linked to Diseases of the Lungs

The ADA and AAE totally dismiss research performed by Weston Price over 90 years ago. In one of his studies, he found that patients with periodontal infections were 2.5 times more likely to develop pneumonia than those who did not have such infections.[66]

Interestingly, a recent study validates Price's finding. It reports that individuals with periodontitis were 2.8 times as likely to develop pneumonia in the hospital (nosocomial pneumonia) as those without periodontal disease.[67] It would appear that Dr. Price was right on the button in his study.

*Individuals with periodontal infections were found to be **five times** more likely to have bronchial inflammation than those without such infections.*

Other investigators report that after providing periodontal treatment to a patient who had experienced many recurrences of chronic lung infections, the patient became free from these recurrences.[68] It has also been noted by medical researchers that dental infections can be an important source for septic pulmonary embolism (an infected blood clot blocking a main artery of the lung).[69]

Chronic obstructive pulmonary disease (COPD) causes progressive damage to lung tissues that results in shortness of breath, cough, and sputum production. Typically, the disease will worsen in stages followed by plateau periods when it seems to remain unchanged. A study clearly linking periodontal infections with worsening COPD found that patients receiving periodontal therapy (not root canal treatment) to remove the infection in the tissues surrounding the tooth experienced a reduced frequency of worsening episodes.[70]

In research showing the relationship between asthma and periodontitis, individuals with periodontal infections were found to be *five times* more likely to have bronchial inflammation than those without such infections.[71] Weston Price reported this correlation as well, as he reported a patient with chronic asthma that cleared up after extraction of five infected teeth.[72]

Periodontitis (and Therefore Root Canal-Treated Teeth) Linked to Diabetes, Obesity, and Metabolic Syndrome

Metabolic syndrome is characterized by a combination of conditions including insulin resistance, hypertension, impaired glucose tolerance or diabetes, raised insulin levels, elevated triglyceride levels, and low levels of high-density cholesterol. It is usually accompanied by abdominal obesity, low energy levels, and fatigue. As a result of these conditions, metabolic syndrome is a well-established risk factor for coronary heart disease. Many studies have linked periodontitis with metabolic syndrome.[73,74,75,76,77,78,79]

This disease is also diagnosed as prediabetes. Other studies also independently link periodontitis with diabetes and obesity.[80,81]

Periodontitis (and Therefore Root Canal-Treated Teeth) Linked to Neurological Problems

Weston Price had much to say about the relationship between infected teeth and maladies of the central nervous system. In discussing this highly prevalent condition he stated, "Our many studies on animals have revealed a definite tendency on the part of the organism, taken from dental infections of patients with central nervous system disturbances, to produce nervous disturbance in rabbits."[82] Price reported on several different neurological conditions, including memory disorders and seizures.

This [root canal-treated] tooth was placed under the skins of 30 consecutive rabbits. All of the rabbits died within 6 days...all of the rabbits developed neurological symptoms... similar to those exhibited by the patient from whom the tooth was extracted.

One such case serves not only as a demonstration of the close relationship between root canal-treated teeth and diseases of the central nervous system, but also as an example of Dr. Price's persistence in demonstrating the reproducibility of his work. In this particular case he extracted a root canal-treated tooth from a patient suffering from a severe disease involving the central nervous system. This tooth was placed under the skins of 30 consecutive rabbits. *All* of the rabbits died within six days. Furthermore, *all* of the rabbits developed neurological symptoms that were similar to those exhibited by the patient from whom the tooth was extracted.[83,84]

In the last few years others have been reporting similar relationships. Periodontitis has been linked to increased severity of epileptic seizures,[85] the possible onset and progression of Alzheimer's disease,[86] and greater neurological deficits in strokes.[87]

Periodontitis (and Therefore Root Canal-Treated Teeth) Linked to Rheumatoid Arthritis

Early in his work, Weston Price linked rheumatoid arthritis with root canal-treated teeth. Although some of his patients showed marked improvement upon extraction of the offending teeth, he readily admitted:

Modern day investigators are now reporting on the periodontitis-arthritis link.

> We have, accordingly, **come to be very guarded in the matter of giving encouragement** for marked relief in all cases of deforming arthritis, because of the seriousness of structural changes, the abundance of the scar tissue (in this case of bony scar tissue), and the permanent susceptibility of such individuals.[88] [emphasis added]

One of the major studies used to "debunk" Price's work, was performed on 52 patients with rheumatoid arthritis who also had root canal-treated teeth. Many wanting to justify the root canal procedure have over-interpreted the results to suggest that since the majority of the patients did not improve upon extraction of the root canal-treated teeth, there is no link between systemic disease and root canal-treated teeth. This fallacious interpretation was addressed earlier in this chapter.

Individuals with periodontitis had a 14% greater risk of developing cancer than those free of periodontitis.

Nevertheless, animals that were injected with cultures from root canal-treated teeth extracted from patients with arthritis frequently developed strikingly similar arthritic deformities. In addition, modern day investigators are now reporting on the periodontitis-arthritis link.[89,90]

Periodontitis (and Therefore Root Canal-Treated Teeth) Linked to Cancer

The origin of many cancers has been traced to sites of infection and inflammation. At the very least, periodontal disease is a chronic inflammatory condition. This inflammation becomes much more serious as the bacteria involved become anaerobic and begin to release toxins. Several investigators have linked dental infections with increased risk of cancer in several tissues,[91] including:

- ✓ Pancreatic cancer[92,93]
- ✓ Lung cancer[94]
- ✓ Gastrointestinal cancer[95]
- ✓ Esophageal and gastric cancers[96]
- ✓ Lip, mouth, tongue, nose, throat, vocal cord, and windpipe cancers[97]
- ✓ Head and neck cancers[98]

In addition to all of these correlations, another study found simply that individuals with periodontitis had a 14% greater risk of developing cancer than those free of periodontitis.[99]

Periodontitis (and Therefore Root Canal-Treated Teeth) Linked to a Host of Other Conditions and Diseases

Justification for the subspecialty called Periodontal Medicine becomes more substantial as researchers continue to uncover more links between periodontal infections and systemic diseases. The following list is not exhaustive but demonstrates the broad correlation between periodontitis and disease. Periodontal infections have been associated with:

- ✓ Low birth weight, pre-term infants, and lower maternal hemoglobin levels[100]
- ✓ Worsened disease activity in systemic lupus erythematosus[101]

✓ Lower hemoglobin levels [102]
✓ Increased risk of preeclampsia [103,104]
✓ Inflammatory bowel disease [105]
✓ Increased cardiac calcification [106]
✓ Bone destruction/resorption (stimulation of osteoclastic activity) [107]
✓ Sudden sensorineural hearing loss [108]
✓ Elevated serum ferritin (iron storage) levels [109]
✓ Ankylosing spondylitis [110]
✓ Psoriasis [111]
✓ Decreased plasma vitamin C levels [112] and vitamin D deficiency [113]

CONCLUSION

Dental professionals claim that there is no scientific evidence that links root canal-treated teeth with systemic disease. They are wrong. The evidence presented in this chapter demonstrates a well-established, clear, and undeniable connection. Regardless of whether the infection is associated with periodontal disease or the deeper bone infection called apical periodontitis, the infecting pathogens and their toxins have been linked to the presence of a wide array of diseases throughout the body.

While the dental industry readily admits some of the health risks associated with these focal periodontal infections, it continues to insist that root canal-treated teeth are unassociated with these links.

Dental professionals claim that, although root canal-treated teeth may host bacteria, this does not prove that these teeth are infected. They are wrong again. Dr. Haley proved otherwise. Root canal-treated teeth do leak very potent exotoxins that directly cause tissue damage and disrupt cellular function. Bacteria present within the root canal-treated tooth produce these toxins.

Anatomical realities, as well as recent scientific studies presented in previous chapters, have shown that all root canal-treated teeth are chronically infected. If the root canal procedure does not introduce new infection into the tooth and jawbone, then the resident infection must still remain because of a failure to eliminate the original infection that was used to justify the root canal procedure in the first place. In addition, the presence of periodontal disease around a root canal-treated tooth will be a source of bacteria to directly enter the dentinal tubules

Many of the systemic disease connections that Dr. Price documented are now being confirmed and published in dental journals.

through the outer cementum layer. Without an intact immune system within the root canal-treated tooth, these bacteria can then easily multiply and release toxins into the body. The root canal-treated tooth also serves as a reservoir to repopulate the periodontal area even after a technically successful treatment for periodontitis has been performed. Over time, then, more and more bacteria can invade the periodontal area and increasing amounts of toxins can be produced.

Price, Rosenow, and others clearly demonstrated the pathogenic nature of infected teeth; many were root canal-treated, others were not. Thousands of rabbits were sacrificed to demonstrate this. The ADA and the AAE have been denying Dr. Price's "long-dispelled theory" for decades at great expense to very many patients. But the truth just won't go away. If these organizations would or could only point to a few published studies that confirm their claim that the vast majority of root canal-treated teeth are free from infection, they could slay this dragon once and for all. They do not because the studies do not exist.

Many of the systemic disease connections that Dr. Price documented are now being confirmed and published in dental journals. Even the medical world is acknowledging the broad-reaching health risks associated with periodontal disease. At a minimum, dental professionals should be required to discuss these established risks and determine, with their patients, whether the benefits of a root canal procedure outweigh the health risks. Quite simply, the root canal procedure requires a fully informed consent explaining all of the potential systemic health risks before the patient decides whether to proceed. To date, this virtually never occurs.

CHAPTER SIX

DEFENSE *of Root Canal Treatment*

The American Association of Endodontists: "The Treatment is Safe"

The American Association of Endodontists (AAE) is an independent member association that exists to protect and promote its members' professional interests. A broad public acceptance of the safety and validity of the root canal procedure is needed in order to justify the AAE's existence. This very reality forces a vehement defense of the root canal procedure and a powerful response against anyone, especially a dental professional, who would call this procedure into question.

That does not imply that everything the AAE does or says is not important or valid, but it does mean that the health needs of dental patients are easily trumped by the organization's self-interest. Actual statements of the AAE have been reproduced below within their context to demonstrate the unscientific bias and even blatant misrepresentation of facts to protect and perpetuate a multi-billion dollar per year industry.

Some of the specific claims made by the AAE have been addressed in previous chapters. To avoid unnecessary redundancy, a more general analysis will follow the position statements that are reproduced here.

AAE Position Statements on Safety of Root Canals

On the 2014 website of the AAE, the safety of the root canal treatment is vigorously asserted. The organization clearly states:

> **There is no valid, scientific evidence linking root canal-treated teeth and disease elsewhere in the body.** A root canal is a safe and effective procedure. When a severe infection in a tooth requires endodontic treatment, that treatment is designed to **eliminate** bacteria from the infected root canal, **prevent** reinfection of the tooth and **save** the natural tooth.[1] [emphasis theirs]

The AAE also asserts that it serves "the best interest of patients to understand there is no valid scientific evidence linking root canals to cancer or other health problems."[1]

The 1994 Fall/Winter AAE informational newsletter addressed the concept that an infection in a localized area (a focal infection), in this case an infected tooth, is tied to systemic disease. On the front page of that newsletter, in large letters, it reads: "Root canal therapy safe and effective." The subsequent text asserts that:

> ...exhaustive and meticulous scientific investigations proved that root canal therapy is a safe and effective means for saving teeth and that endodontically treated teeth do not serve as foci for infection in other parts of the body.[2]

Another article in the same newsletter is entitled: "When infection does spread from an infected root canal." In it the author concludes:

> In the case of the acute periradicular [apical periodontitis] abscess, infection from the root canal spreads to immediately adjacent structures in the periapex [around the tooth root] and then to immediately adjacent fascial [connective tissue] spaces of the head and neck, resulting in cellulitis [bacterial skin infection] and systemic signs of infection. This is not an example of focal infection, where bacterial travel through the circulatory system and establish infection at a site distant from the focus of infection.[3]

It is well-documented that subacute bacterial endocarditis can come from infected teeth or gums.

The above statement is absurd. How can the AAE state with authority that an infection from a root canal-treated tooth will always stay put locally around the tooth and never disseminate to the rest of the body? It is not a medically sound statement, and it defies simple logic. *Of course* an infection can spread to other places in the body. It is well-documented that sub-acute bacterial endocarditis can come from infected teeth or gums, which are foci of oral infection. A similar example is the brain abscess that is caused by a dental infection. It is clear that the AAE is not telling the whole truth.

AAE Position Statement on Toxin Dissemination

In the early 1950's a Swiss dentist by the name of Angelo Sargenti began to use an alternative to gutta-percha to fill root canal-treated teeth. This filler was a paste that contained paraformaldehyde. In 1991 the AAE issued a strong statement against the use of this chemical in the root canal procedure:

> Paraformaldehyde-containing endodontic filling materials or sealers (frequently known as Sargenti pastes, N-2, N-2 Universal, RC-2B or RC-2B White) should not be used for endodontic treatment because those materials are unsafe. Extensive scientific research has proven unequivocally that paraformaldehyde-containing filling materials and sealers can cause irreversible damage to tissues near the root canal system including the following: destruction of connective tissue and bone; intractable pain; paresthesia and dysthesia of the mandibular and maxillary nerves; and chronic infections of the maxillary sinus. ***Moreover, scientific evidence has demonstrated that the damage from paraformalde-***

hyde-containing filling materials and sealers is not necessarily confined to tissues near the root canal. The active ingredients of these filling materials and sealers have been found to travel throughout the body and have been shown to infiltrate the blood, lymph nodes, adrenal glands, kidney, spleen, liver and brain.[4]
(emphasis ours)

This AAE statement about paraformalde-hyde-containing root canal filling materials admits that scientific research demonstrates that the para-formaldehyde contained in such materials does not stay confined to the tissues near the root canal. This is true and the warning is justified. However, if paraformaldehyde can infiltrate the blood, lymph nodes, adrenal glands, kidney, spleen, liver, and brain from a root canal-treated tooth, then there is nothing to keep bacteria and their associated toxins that reside in the same tooth from infiltrating into those systems and organs throughout the body as well.

If paraformaldehyde can disseminate systemically, bacterial toxins most certainly disseminate as well.

Systemic dissemination of toxic dental chemicals is not somehow magically limited to paraformaldehyde. The bacterial toxins noted above readily enter the blood and lymphatic circulations, and they easily pass through tissue membranes making systemic dissemination a certainty. If paraformaldehyde can disseminate systemically, bacterial toxins most certainly disseminate as well.

AAE Position Statements Against Tooth Extraction

In a section about root canal treatment "myths" on the AAE website regarding the subject of extraction as an option to a root canal procedure, the organization states:

> **Saving your natural teeth, if possible, is the very best option.**
> Nothing can completely replace your natural tooth. An artificial tooth can sometimes cause you to avoid certain foods. Keeping your own teeth is important so that you can continue to enjoy the wide variety of foods necessary to maintain the proper nutrient balance in your diet. If your dentist recommends extraction, ask whether root canal treatment is an option.
>
> Endodontic [root canal] treatment, along with appropriate restoration, is a cost-effective way to treat teeth with damaged pulp and is usually less expensive than extraction and placement of a bridge or an implant.
>
> **Endodontic treatment also has a very high success rate. Many root canal-treated teeth last a lifetime.**
> Placement of a bridge or an implant will require significantly more time in treatment and may result in further procedures to adjacent teeth and supporting tissues.

Millions of healthy endodontically treated teeth serve patients all over the world, years and years after treatment. Those healthy teeth are helping patients chew efficiently, maintain the natural appearance of their smiles and enhance their enjoyment of life. Through endodontic treatment, endodontists and dentists worldwide enable patients to keep their natural teeth for a lifetime.[1] (emphasis theirs)

AAE Position Statements Examined

Several claims in the AAE statements can be proven false. Six of these will be addressed one at a time.

1. **"There is no valid, scientific evidence linking root canal-treated teeth and disease elsewhere in the body."[1]**

    In most cases the reason for performing a root canal procedure on a tooth is because it is infected. This infection is diagnosed by patient symptoms, X-ray evaluation, or both. Chapter Five cites scores of "valid, scientific" studies that "link" periodontitis (infection of the jawbone around the tooth root) to a long list of systemic diseases. As we have shown, apical periodontitis associated with a root canal-treated tooth as well as the tooth itself can have similar adverse systemic health effects.

    The appearance of "periodontitis" around root canal-treated teeth has been used to determine the failure rates of this procedure in a number of large "valid, scientific" dental studies (documented in Chapter Three).

If a tooth with periodontal disease is linked to systemic diseases, then a root canal-treated tooth with apical periodontitis is linked to the same diseases.

The two dimensional X-ray diagnosed infection rate in root canal-treated teeth was as high as 64.5%. Conventional X-rays fail to show an additional 20% or more of these infections due to technical limitations. A huge percentage of root canal-treated teeth are nevertheless demonstrably infected, while others are infected but simply undetected by X-ray.

These periodontal infections have been linked to systemic diseases by a number of "valid, scientific" studies (see Chapter Five). If a tooth with periodontal disease is linked to systemic diseases, then a root canal-treated tooth with apical periodontitis is liked to the same diseases.

The fact that the root canal treatment fails to eliminate infection establishes its relation to systemic disease. But, the infected root canal-treated tooth is potentially even more dangerous because it allows the infection to proliferate, often without detection, as long as the tooth remains in the mouth, and the act of chewing on such a tooth generates very high pressures, pushing pathogens and toxins directly into the venous and lymphatic drainage pathways in the jawbone.

2. **"As recently as 2013, research published in *JAMA Otolaryngology—Head & Neck Surgery*, found that patients with multiple endodontic treatments had a 45 percent reduced risk of cancer."** [5]

    The AAE has used one handpicked artifact from this study to mislead readers to a false conclusion. This is a very deceptive for a couple of reasons:

    ✓ The study was performed to "test the association between dental caries and head and neck squamous cell carcinoma (HNSCC)" not to determine the impact of root canal-treated teeth on the incidence of cancer. Test subjects were divided into thirds based on the incidence of dental caries (cavities). Of the top third of those with cavities who had undergone root canal treatments, 45% had less incidence of HNSCC. Interestingly, those with three or more cavities had 68% less incidence of HNSCC.

    Multiple root canal treatments were seen as objective measures of a long-standing history of cavities. The researchers' only stated conclusion: "There is an inverse association between HNSCC and dental caries." In other words, the more cavities, the lower the incidence of HNSCC. Using the AAE's logic, people could reduce their risk of getting HNSCC by engaging in activities that would produce more cavities.

✓ A particular type of cancer (head and neck squamous cell carcinoma) was the only cancer investigated. There are many types of cancer. Just because subjects with multiple root canal-treated teeth were found to have a lower incidence of one very specialized cancer, does not mean that root canal treatment is associated in any way with an overall lower incidence of cancer throughout the body.

Science should be the complete and objective reporting of the facts after evaluation of ALL the data and should never show bias.

What is even more disturbing is that the AAE put this article on their website while **NEVER** putting any of the numerous studies listed in this book that show the negative health impact of root canal-treated teeth. Science should be the complete and objective reporting of the facts after evaluation of **ALL** the data and should never show bias. Selectively picking articles that are favorable to a position, while omitting all negative articles is not science. Any organization that does so can no longer be considered a scientific organization, but rather a biased and ideologically self-serving group.

3. **"...exhaustive and meticulous scientific investigations proved that root canal therapy is a safe and effective procedure."**[1]

Considering the fact that dentists performing root canal procedures have been fighting the concept of the dissemination of focal infection for nearly 100 years, it would seem logical that if research "proving" the safety of the treatment did in fact exist, it would be front and center. Of all the studies listed on the AAE website, none of them prove, or even claim to prove, anything, much less the safety of the root canal procedure.

Three recent studies... show that individuals who have undergone root canal treatment are more likely to have coronary heart disease.

It is true that hundreds of millions of these procedures have been performed in the last 100 years and that there is little, if any, evidence that significant numbers of people have succumbed as a direct result of the procedure. However, it is not "proof" that a treatment is without health risk if a proper scientific study is never performed.

In fact, three recent studies, one that was published in the *Journal of the American Dental Association*, were cited in the last chapter to show that individuals who have undergone root canal treatment are more likely to have coronary heart disease than those who haven't had any root canal treatments. If a dental procedure increases the incidence of a deadly disease, is it really safe?

4. **"When infection does spread from an infected root canal... In the case of the acute periradicular abscess, infection from the root canal spreads to immediately adjacent structures in the periapex and then immediately adjacent fascial spaces of the head and neck, resulting in cellulitis and systemic signs and symptoms of infection. This is not an example of focal infection, where bacteria travel through the circulatory system and establish infection at a site distant from the focus of infection."[3]**

    Although this statement is not untrue on its face, its unstated purpose is to make the claim that apical periodontitis is not an example of a focal infection. Yes, the infection does first spread to the tissues immediately adjacent to the root canal-treated tooth. This is true. But what they fail to state is that this infection, like any other infection in the body, can also enter the circulatory system and be spread systemically. Making the statement that this infection can only remain adjacent to the tooth is completely false and misleading. And the lymphatic and venous drainage at the apex of the tooth makes such spread even easier.

Research confirms the migration of periodontitis-associated bacteria through the circulatory system. As cited in Chapter Five, bacterial DNA "typical for endodontic infection" has been found buried in the arterial walls of patients with coronary heart disease and blood clots aspirated from the blocked arteries of heart attack victims. Since both the clots and the plaques reside in the circulatory system, it seems clear that pathogens from anywhere around the tooth can be disseminated via this pathway.

5. **"Saving your natural teeth, if possible, is the very best option."**[1]

This statement assumes overall health is not an important issue. If health is not an issue, then the claim is true. For some, the ***appearance*** of a mouth full of healthy teeth seems to be more important than actual health, especially in the younger generation.

However, when overall quality of life and economics are considered, a bridge, implant, partial denture, or perhaps even a missing tooth is preferable to a stroke, heart attack, cancer, arthritis, dementia, diabetes, and other systemic diseases. Links from infected teeth to each of these conditions have been demonstrated in the scientific literature. Causality has not been proven, but neither has any study proved that these infections are not involved in the initiation or worsening of these diseases.

> *Patients are rarely told of the possible health risks prior to [root canal] treatment, and therefore are not really given the opportunity to make an informed choice.*

Throughout all of the medical literature causality is rarely proven, as costly large prospective studies are generally required to establish this. And even though an established link does not mean cause-and-effect, the resolution of a disease by removing an established link or risk factor is, in fact, compelling evidence for a cause-and-effect relationship.

Unfortunately, patients are rarely told of the possible health risks prior to treatment, and therefore are not really given the opportunity to make an informed choice.

6. **"Endodontic treatment also has a very high success rate. Many root canal-treated teeth last a lifetime."**[1]

Several root canal treatment evaluation studies cited in Chapter Three report "success" rates between 39%-59%. These figures are based on the observation of periapical lesions with two-dimensional X-rays. Three-dimensional X-rays reduce those "proofs" of success by about another 30%. Depending upon one's definition of "very high success rate" this may or may not be acceptable.

A root canal-treated tooth is hollow and porous. Endodontists believe that these teeth contain a filling and sealer that makes them harmless. Substantial research shows that such teeth contain pathogens and toxins which continually leak out of the inside of the tooth, and are far from harmless. If the research showing that root canal-treated teeth are still infected is valid, the fact that such a tooth remains in the mouth is cause for serious concern.

The Danger of Professional Organizations Like the ADA and the AAE

The mere size of the ADA and its specialty organization, the AAE, both in terms of membership and money, gives them policy clout that is not necessarily merited. These groups are advocates for their constituent members, *not* advocates for patient rights or health *per se*, and yet they are perceived as credible and even altruistic, all the while aggressively promoting procedures that arguably present systemic health risks to those patients subjected to them.

If the Food and Drug Administration (FDA) was diligently guarding the public health, the available scientific evidence on the safety of the root canal procedure would compel them to require a prominent display of a disclaimer that might read...

WARNING: This procedure may be hazardous to your health. Research has shown that it may increase your risk for heart disease, lung disease, kidney disease, dementia, diabetes, and arthritis.

Any dentist or endodontist reading this can breathe a sigh of relief. The FDA has shown no interest in this major threat to public health, and it is unlikely they will ever require such disclosure, even with intense public pressure. But, if they did, much of the multi-billion dollar dental industry would be decimated overnight. And that's precisely why we believe that the ADA and AAE work so hard to quell any notion that root canal treatment may actually pose a significant health risk.

Because the ADA and AAE wield such powerful political lobbies, they pose an even more insidious risk. When a position statement appears in one of their professional newsletters or on one of their websites, it tends to become an accepted standard of care.

Dental professionals who deviate from the stated position do so at their own peril. Such deviation, regardless of the potential benefit to the patient, can be considered misconduct by the state dental boards, and the dentist can be brought up on such charges. In these cases, there is no fair trial, no benefit of a substantive defense, and no opportunity to present scientific studies that justify the dentist's actions. Dental licensing boards set the rules. They have unquestioned and unlimited authority to penalize dentists who deviate from the standard of care, and they can revoke licenses as they see fit. A license to practice dentistry is considered a privilege, not a right. Therefore, "standard of care" is determined by the profession itself, and any dental board prosecution does not permit the rights accorded in the constitutional court system.

This reality suggests some important questions:

✓ Who is examining the important relationship between dental health and
overall systemic health?

✓ Who is reviewing the literature to see if
what the ADA, AAE, or anyone else says
is true or not?

✓ How can a patient be sure that any given
dental procedure will not cause disease
somewhere else in the body?

Unfortunately, **no one's minding the store!**
What's worse, as in so many arenas, there is little
or no tolerance for a dissenting voice—regardless
of evidence, experience, or logical validity. A thinking dentist who is legitimately concerned about his
patients' health can quickly find himself or herself unemployed and even unemployable (see the
Preface). It is not likely that this book will change
the status quo regarding dental procedures in the
near future, but it is hoped that it will provide the
ammunition necessary for individuals to make
informed decisions and to insist on the optimal dental care for themselves and their families.

CHAPTER SEVEN

CASE HISTORIES *of Root Canal Treatment*

Clear and Present Danger

Personal & Professional Experience of Robert Kulacz, DDS

Admittedly, personal observations by one dentist are insufficient proof of anything. However, many years of training and practice as a dentist have provided numerous confirmations of the dangers associated with the root canal procedure that have been substantiated by many researchers through the years. I recount a few of those many experiences here to further demonstrate the health risks associated with root canal-treated teeth.

In addition, these accounts serve as examples of the refusal by many of my colleagues in the medical and dental professions to accept needed changes in long accepted practices in spite of the abundance of past and present evidence that more than justifies such changes.

Fellow Students "Altering" Procedures

When I was taught to do root canal procedures in dental school the importance of sterilizing the root canal space was emphasized. This was deemed so important by the dental professors that we were required to take a specimen for culture from the inside of the root canal and send it to the lab to see if any bacteria would grow. Only when the culture came back negative, meaning that there was no growth of bacteria from the specimen, were we allowed to finish the root canal procedure.

They would often fake this test by placing a sterile collecting swab into the culture media without actually taking a sample from the root canal space in the tooth being treated.

During the time of my training, many students became frustrated because the culture results kept coming back positive. Because of this, they would often fake this test by placing a sterile collecting swab into the culture media without actually taking a sample from the root canal space in the tooth being treated. This way a negative culture would be guaranteed, and they could then finish the root canal procedure.

But even if the students were conscientious and eventually submitted samples that showed no growth, this was no assurance that the tooth was sterile. For one thing, most of the bacteria infecting root canal-treated teeth are anaerobic, meaning that they cannot live or grow in the presence of oxygen.

These anaerobic bacteria have to be cultured using specific techniques not ordinarily employed. Some of these bacteria are very slow growing and need to be incubated for up to two weeks to see growth, longer than the normal two to three days as was the procedure at the time. So, even if the culture came back negative, it would be useless in predicting whether the root canal-treated tooth was infected with the more commonly present anaerobic bacteria.

Even if the culture came back negative, it would be useless in predicting whether the root canal-treated tooth was infected with the more commonly present anaerobic bacteria.

Extracted Root Canal-Treated Teeth Fail to Pass the "Smell" Test

When I was still a practicing dentist, I would often have occasion to extract root canal-treated teeth. The indications for the extractions were because X-ray revealed periapical infections or because the teeth were only being extracted as part of an orthodontic treatment protocol (braces). Removal of these root canal-treated teeth was always an enlightening event for the patient having the extraction.

If a patient was not completely convinced of the need for extraction before the procedure, that quickly changed afterward. I made it a point to show the extracted tooth to the patient. Many times it was discolored, with infected tissue around the tip of the root. I would also show them the mushy or discolored diseased bone that I removed from the extraction socket.

My dental assistant once described an extracted root canal-treated tooth as smelling like a dead mouse that had been decomposing for a while.

But the most convincing moment came when I let the curious patient smell the extracted tooth. With a predicable jolt, the patient's head would turn to the side. The odor of dead and infected tissue is an unforgettable smell. My dental assistant once described an extracted root canal-treated tooth as smelling like a dead mouse that had been decomposing for a while.

By contrast, healthy teeth extracted for reasons such as braces have normal color and no foul odor. They are not infected, and therefore have no associated dead and rotting tissue.

Cause of Death: A Root Canal-Treated Tooth?

Mr. Smith's condition was deteriorating rapidly. It had been a month since his shortness of breath forced him to be admitted to the hospital. His family was gathered in a conference room along with two of his physicians.

The pulmonologist (lung specialist) spoke to the group: "We do not have any answers as to the cause of Mr. Smith's condition. We looked everywhere for a primary source for the infection but we found nothing."

At that point I felt compelled to speak up. "No you didn't. You didn't check his mouth. Mr. Smith has two root canals and moderate to severe gum disease."

The pulmonologist appeared to completely ignore my comment, although his quick glance at the cardiologist sitting in the corner appeared to be an attempt to see if he had support in regarding my suggestion as ludicrous. At the time, the oral-systemic disease link was not much discussed in the dental and medical professions, and it was very clear to me that this physician was not willing to even entertain the possibility of an oral focus as the cause of Mr. Smith's condition. Unfortunately, Mr. Smith died the next day.

With the family's permission I obtained Mr. Smith's complete hospital record. There were more question marks and frustrated uncertainties in the chart than there were definitive answers. It seemed that nobody had any idea why Mr. Smith was sick.

And, still, there was no diagnosis. There was never a diagnosis.

Certainly, nobody put into writing any scientifically plausible hypothesis as to why Mr. Smith was so sick.

Multiple consultations by a variety of medical specialists led to the same diagnostic dead-end. Even though his blood tests indicated that Mr. Smith had a bacterial infection, blood cultures for bacteria were negative. Lacking any clear answers for his condition, the treating physicians tried one antibiotic after another.

This non-focused, machine gun-like administration of multiple drugs continued until Mr. Smith's kidneys and liver could no longer handle the toxic assault of these drugs along with the toxic effects of his underlying disease. Faced with this relentless toxicity and the ongoing stress of the unchecked infection, these organs finally began to shut down. And, still, there was no diagnosis. There was never a diagnosis. The question marks continued to pile up in the medical record.

Mr. Smith, however, is not such an unusual case. Many people die every day in hospitals without a clear diagnosis. The final cause of death in such a patient commonly ends up being the "diagnosis," such as heart attack, blood clot, stroke, or respiratory failure. But what led up to so many of these "final causes" of death?

Sixteen years before his death, Mr. Smith had a root canal procedure on one of his teeth. During this treatment process he developed a heart infection known as subacute bacterial endocarditis (SBE). Bacteria from his infected, root canal-treated tooth entered the bloodstream and traveled to Mr. Smith's heart. SBE is often a life-threatening illness. Although an infected tooth is not the only source of the bacteria or other microorganisms that can cause SBE, Mr. Smith's SBE was clearly traced to his root canal-treated tooth.

These pathogens invaded and grew upon one of the heart valves. The damage to the heart valve was so severe that it became necessary to do a heart valve replacement surgery. Mr. Smith still had that same root canal-treated tooth in his mouth in addition to others, and he had moderate to severe periodontal disease.

> *During this [root canal] treatment process he developed a heart infection known as subacute bacterial endocarditis.*

This raised a very significant and logical question: After already having had such a severe illness caused by a dental infection, why wasn't the possibility of disease-provoking oral bacteria explored as a cause for Mr. Smith's current illness?

Just as a chronic infection anywhere else in the body would have clinical significance in a medical work-up, the mouth should be no different. Instead the ADA insists that root canal-treated teeth can never cause or contribute to any systemic disease and is somehow the magical exception to accepted medical principles. As long as the root canal procedure is viewed as a "sacred" treatment that is beyond question, people will suffer and some will needlessly die.

Case: Root Canal Toxins Nearly Fatal

A root canal procedure is judged to be a success when the pain has gone away and the bone around the root that was previously involved with the infection appears healed on X-ray examination.

Most endodontists will perform a root canal procedure on any tooth that is technically treatable by the procedure regardless of the degree of infection or of the virulence and disease-causing capabilities of the microbes that are involved. In fact, a grossly infected tooth is one of the primary reasons that many root canal procedures are performed. The endodontist actually believes that the root canal procedure can sometimes eliminate the infection in such a tooth, and that any remaining bacteria will remain safely entombed within the tooth.

I observed this first-hand when a physician in my town had a problem with a root canal-treated tooth. This physician had a root canal procedure started on a front tooth on a Thursday. By Saturday he was in so much pain that he called his endodontist back.

Endodontists seldom recommend extraction of any tooth that they consider "restorable," no matter how infected it may be. This physician's endodontist agreed to see him that morning, and proceeded to lightly instrument and irrigate the root canal space.

On his way home, the physician began to feel extremely ill.

On his way home, the physician began to feel extremely ill. He told his wife to drive him to the hospital emergency room.

He told his wife to drive him to the hospital emergency room. Upon arrival he was barely lucid. He was running a high fever, his heart rate was above 160 beats per minute, and his blood pressure was dangerously low.

He kept pleading with the emergency room staff not to let him die. The doctor was then admitted to the intensive care unit in a state of shock. The infectious disease specialists began treating him with antibiotics. The antibiotics they chose were primarily useful in killing aerobic bacteria, which are bacteria that thrive in the presence of oxygen.

However, these drugs were not effective against the bacteria inside the root canal-treated tooth, since those bacteria were living in an oxygen-deprived environment and were anaerobic bacteria. Furthermore, the tooth no longer had a viable blood supply since the pulp was removed in the root canal procedure. This made it impossible for even the correct antibiotic to get inside the tooth where the infection persisted. Therefore, the antibiotics administered were of no use in fighting this infection. More importantly, it was the extremely potent toxins that the bacteria produced that were introduced into the bloodstream just a few hours before—during the instrumentation of the root canal space—that caused the toxic shock.

It was the extremely potent toxins that the bacteria produced that were introduced into the bloodstream just a few hours before—during the instrumentation of the root canal space—that caused the toxic shock.

Antibiotics can only affect the bacteria directly. Antibiotics have no effect at all on the toxins that these bacteria have already produced. Neither the physicians nor the attending dentists were familiar with the oral bacteria and their pathogenicity in an oxygen-starved environment. Fortunately, this particular patient was an otherwise healthy young man with a relatively strong immune system. He was released from the intensive care unit after three days of being extremely ill with no apparent permanent damage.

Had he been older or more immunologically compromised the outcome would likely not have been so favorable. But younger and stronger immune systems will often make clinical mismanagement look like appropriate, or at least acceptable, care.

It would now seem logical that you should have a tooth that nearly killed you extracted as soon as possible. In fact, that is what I recommended. However, I received a call from an oral surgeon on the hospital staff who felt that the tooth

It would now seem logical that you should have a tooth that nearly killed you extracted as soon as possible.

could be saved by completing the root canal procedure. He stated that we had to try and save this tooth since this physician was a prominent member of the medical staff and the community.

The physician's primary dentist also felt that the tooth could, and should, be "saved" and not extracted. In the face of these identical recommendations the physician decided not to extract the tooth but instead to complete the root canal procedure and keep the tooth. As mentioned earlier, there are few endodontists who would recommend extraction of any clinically restorable tooth regardless of the toxicity contained within.

Meanwhile, the same bacteria that nearly killed the physician earlier remained within the porous dentinal tubules of his root canal-treated tooth, continually producing and releasing the same toxins into his body. His next illness only awaits the eventual inability of his immune system to keep on fighting this chronic infection and to keep on neutralizing the potent bacterial toxins being released. That failure of the immune system may take days, weeks, months, and sometimes years.

Furthermore, this chronic toxicity and inflammation coupled with other risk factors will often present as a life-threatening disease such as a heart attack, or even as the ultimate disease of immune failure, cancer.

When such a disease occurs years after the root canal procedure was performed, the appropriate correlation between this procedure and the onset of the disease is rarely made. As a result, the root canal-treated tooth remains in the jawbone, and the chronic infection and toxin production in that tooth continues.

Myocarditis Resolves After Root Canal-Treated Teeth Extracted— Heart Transplant No Longer Necessary

I had treated a patient who was in severe heart failure and scheduled for a heart transplant. He was referred to me prior to heart transplant surgery to clear all oral infections. He had several root canal-treated teeth and severe periodontal disease with infection spreading into the maxillary sinus. I extracted the infected teeth, curetted out the associated granulation tissue and infected bone, and curetted the diseased tissue from the floor of the maxillary sinus. The infection within the maxillary sinus was severe with purulent drainage in both the sinus and the jawbone.

Soon after, his ejection fraction improved to the point that a heart transplant was no longer indicated.

After receiving the microbiological culture results, I put him on the antibiotics shown to be effective against these bacteria. Soon after, his ejection fraction improved to the point that a heart transplant was no longer indicated. This patient undoubtedly had at least some degree of myocarditis acutely compromising contractility, and it was suspected that the toxin/infection removal allowed a sufficient amount of the inflamed myocardium to recover.

"Seeing is Denying" — Restored Health Upon Extraction of Infected Teeth Deemed "Coincidence"

Elizabeth was a 33-year-old female of normal height and weight with no history of any significant medical problems. One day she began having pain in the right kidney area. Her symptoms escalated to bouts of vomiting and diarrhea. Elizabeth's blood pressure was severely elevated, she was rapidly losing weight, and she was suffering from extreme fatigue.

Elizabeth's internist was concerned enough about her clinical appearance that she was then admitted to the hospital. Medications were given to control her blood pressure, and antibiotics were given to fight the apparent kidney infection. Although Elizabeth showed slight improvement while in the hospital, she continued to have pain in her right kidney area. She was also having difficulty keeping food down, and she continued to lose weight. Her doctors told her that it would take at least six months for her to get better and that there was nothing more that they could do. She was released from the hospital and was monitored as an outpatient.

> *When Elizabeth arrived in my office her general appearance was poor. She was extremely thin with a pale complexion, and she could barely walk into the treatment room without feeling exhausted.*

Instead of getting better, Elizabeth got worse. Her family did not know what to do. The doctors did not seem to have an answer, and Elizabeth's health continued its rapid decline.

Elizabeth's mother heard from a relative about my work with infected teeth and their effect on general health. Although they had their doubts about how a tooth could cause such a serious medical condition they felt that they were at the end of the road and that no other medical options remained. Elizabeth and her family felt at this point that anything was worth a try.

When Elizabeth arrived in my office her general appearance was poor. She was extremely thin with a pale complexion, and she could barely walk into the treatment room without feeling exhausted. After a thorough medical history, I did a dental exam.

The dental exam showed that Elizabeth had one infected root canal-treated tooth and two other infected molars. Although she had no pain associated with these teeth, both the clinical exam and the X-ray exam confirmed the infection. It is always extremely important to evaluate all of the teeth under such circumstances, not just those that are painful.

When the immune system has been chronically weakened by a root canal-treated tooth, other infected teeth will sometimes not be clinically apparent. Remember that inflammation and pus production are indicators that the immune system is doing its job. Lack of these signs can just mean that the immune system needs to be unburdened before it can recover enough to react appropriately against other sub-clinically infected teeth.

Elizabeth then had the relationship between infected teeth and the rest of the body explained to her. She was told that if she were to go to her physicians with an infection on her hand of the same severity as was present in her teeth, it would receive top priority as a possible cause of her medical condition. But because physicians are not trained to look for dental disease as a cause for disease elsewhere in the body they did not even consider this possibility. And, of course, most dentists feel that dental disease is confined to the mouth only. This perspective has somewhat changed since *The Roots of Disease* was published in 2002, but the change is confined to the links between systemic diseases and periodontitis, not to root canal-treated teeth.

Although the importance of having the infected teeth removed was stressed, Elizabeth could not be guaranteed that they were causing her present condition. Another undiagnosed, non-dental infection could still be at least part of the reason for her illness. Nevertheless, Elizabeth elected to have the infected teeth removed.

Within days Elizabeth began to feel better. Two weeks after the extractions she went back to her physician. The physician found that Elizabeth's blood pressure had returned to normal, and the high blood pressure medication being administered to Elizabeth was discontinued. When Elizabeth explained to her doctor that she had three infected teeth removed and asked him if that could have been the source of her problem, he said that it was "only a coincidence" and that the extraction of the teeth had nothing to do with her improvement. Even when these dental reasons for diseases are literally staring some physicians and dentists in their faces, awareness of this critical and common link between medicine and dentistry remains rarely appreciated.

Within one month Elizabeth gained back all of her weight plus five pounds more. She said she was feeling fantastic. Before the extraction of the infected teeth Elizabeth's health had continued to decline for months. After the extractions her health immediately improved.

> *Before the extraction of the infected teeth Elizabeth's health had continued to decline for months. After the extractions her health immediately improved.*

The connection between the mouth and the rest of the body was indisputable in Elizabeth's case. Yet medical schools and dental schools do not teach these important associations, so they remain unknown to most physicians and dentists for the entirety of their professional careers, while many other "Elizabeths" continue to "slip through the cracks." And now, in 2014, the medical and dental schools still do not teach about the important connections between the mouth and the rest of the body.

Personal Observation: Nearly All Root Canal-Treated Teeth Are Still Infected

I have found that nearly all root canal-treated teeth that I have extracted still contain remnants of necrotic pulp tissue and are incompletely sealed by the root canal filling material. This was determined by microscopic examination. How could it be any different? The root canal procedure in which the pulp tissue is cleaned from the root canal space is an imprecise and blind procedure at best. There is no conceivable way that this evacuation of pulp tissue, especially in curved and divergent root canal systems, can ensure complete removal of all infected pulp tissue.

Pathology reports from extracted root canal-treated teeth also typically reflect the presence of infected and dead tissue that had never been completely removed from the main, central canal inside the tooth.

Furthermore, a significant portion of the area targeted for evacuation is physically far beyond the reach of the root canal instruments. And even if the pulp tissue was somehow 100% removed, the instruments cannot clean the miles of the surrounding infected dentinal tubules that always harbor bacteria when the pulp is infected.

And as has been discussed in Chapter Five, even a potentially sterile root canal-treated tooth will soon become infected without the positive fluid flow present in a vital tooth pushing outward through the dentinal tubules and preventing an influx of bacteria. The infection also takes hold since there is no longer a sufficient immune presence remaining in the tooth.

Pathology reports from extracted root canal-treated teeth also typically reflect the presence of infected and dead tissue that had never been completely removed from the main, central canal inside the tooth. Therefore, if we know that even the *most accessible* internal part of the tooth cannot be completely cleaned in most cases, it is obvious that the main bulk of the tooth surrounding this canal that is *not accessible* during a

Although pain can be an indicator of infection, the lack of pain is no assurance that a chronic, low-grade infection is not present.

root canal procedure must always remain infected. This part of the tooth is comprised of the laterally radiating accessory canals and the innumerable, microscopic dentinal tubules. This further establishes that the purported goal of a root canal procedure, the elimination of bacteria and infection, can never be obtained.

Since the actual elimination of bacteria in the tooth is never really achieved, most endodontists can only hope that the bacteria have been eradicated. An X-ray can never detect the chronic harboring of bacteria in the dentinal tubules along with the metabolic toxins that they continually produce.

However, as has been now shown in 3D X-ray imaging, even if there is evidence of bone healing on 2D X-ray, most root canal-treated teeth continue to have demonstrable periapical pathology at the apical foramen. Toxins produced and released from bacteria within the root canal-treated tooth will never make a shadow on an X-ray. Furthermore, although pain can be an indicator of infection, the lack of pain is no assurance that a chronic, low-grade infection is not present.

As described earlier, pain is not always present, even in the most toxic of root canal-treated teeth. In fact, as already mentioned, the root canal canal-treated teeth that have the least discomfort and associated symptoms can be the most toxic. Just as in the example of women with infected tampons and toxic shock syndrome, severely toxic and even fatal consequences can occur in the absence of pain at the site of toxin production. In toxic shock syndrome this site is the infected tampon, and in the dental patient this site is the root canal-treated tooth.

Endodontists Refuse to Answer Legitimate Questions

Two prominent dentists who were members of a New York endodontic group attended a lecture that I gave. At this event, they attempted to refute most of the scientific data presented with unscientific information. They were also offered a significant collection of clinical data on root canal-treated teeth but refused to accept it for review. Later I re-contacted these same two dentists and faxed them a copy of the following questions.

1) What is the goal of a root canal procedure?
2) Can bacteria remain in ideally treated root canal teeth?
3) Can bacteria or bacterial toxins be released from ideally treated root canal teeth?
4) Can ideally treated root canal teeth cause or contribute to systemic disease?
5) Is there any medical contraindication to a root canal procedure?
6) Is there any clinically restorable tooth on which you would not perform a root canal? If so, what would be the basis for your decision?
7) What is the indication for an apicoectomy and what are you trying to achieve with this procedure?

The doctors never did respond. No replies to the questions or return phone calls were ever received.

After about three weeks without a reply, several phone calls were placed to their office. The response of the receptionist was always the same: "The doctor is unavailable and busy with patients but will call you back." The doctors never did respond. No replies to the questions or return phone calls were ever received.

These seven questions were also officially presented to the AAE. An employee of the AAE, who identified herself as the public and professional affairs coordinator of the AAE, had one of the AAE dentists deal with this inquiry. Over the phone, this dentist was informed that a book on the root canal procedure was being written, and the official position of the AAE on several issues was being sought. He responded that he would be glad to help, and he stated that he had the authority to speak directly for the AAE. He requested that the questions be faxed to him and that he would reply in about a week.

A return call was finally received from a lady who identified herself as an assistant director of the AAE. She said that the AAE was refusing to comment on the seven questions that were presented!

When no follow-up phone call from this dentist was received, he was re-contacted. He now asked what the intentions of the book were. He was advised that the book was aimed at informing the public about the truth regarding root canal procedures. He said that the board of directors at the AAE had some legal issues to work out before the questions could be answered.

Again a follow-up call was promised for the following week. And again, no call was received. After attempting one more time to contact him, a message was left, and a return call was finally received from a lady who identified herself as an assistant director of the AAE. She said that the AAE was refusing to comment on the seven questions that were presented! She even commented, "The AAE is not here to help you write a book." After she said that the AAE would freely supply such information to the general public, she was told that this was an inquiry from a member of the public and that answers were being sought regarding the AAE's declared area of expertise. She continued to decline comment and the conversation ended abruptly. What are these dentists and the American Association of Endodontics so afraid of?

Every patient scheduled for a root canal procedure should be advised to ask their dentist these seven questions. Also, seek the answers directly from the AAE. In addition, the AAE has no scientific article to refute the work of Weston Price and E.C. Rosenow, although they claim that they do. None of the articles offered by the AAE effectively disproves the focal infection concept or the negative health effects of root canal-treated teeth.

You have a right to know the answers. It just might be tough to know which answers are correct. Demand to see the scientific evidence for all of the answers you are given. If such evidence is not forthcoming, be suspicious and more demanding, not less.

CHAPTER EIGHT

EXPERIENCE *with Root Canal Treatment*

Before My Own Eyes

Personal & Professional Experience of
Thomas E. Levy, MD, JD

Storybook Perfect—Almost

Thirty years ago I was just a "regular" cardiologist and a non-discriminating consumer of whatever the dental profession deemed most appropriate for treating whatever dental problem I might have had.

I had an adult cardiology practice in New Iberia, Louisiana after finishing up my training at the then-thriving Charity Hospital of New Orleans (never to re-open after Hurricane Katrina in 2005), Tulane University "division." Charity Hospital had always been split 50-50 between the medical students, interns, residents, and fellows of Tulane Medical School on its eastern side, and the LSU Medical School on its western side. It actually made for a very vibrant and lively learning and living experience.

When I finally departed New Orleans for New Iberia, I was ready to start saving patients and continuing the enjoyment of my life to its fullest. I can't say that I had any regrets over just about anything in my life between entering medical school in 1972 and practicing cardiology in New Iberia until 1991. I truly felt sorry for so many of my colleagues who seem so stressed out during their medical school and post-graduate training, and then during their high-volume private practices. I had nothing but fun. I felt blessed.

A Tiny Piece of Bone and a Root Canal

About 5 years into my practice in New Iberia, I bit into a piece of bone in a hamburger that I was eating. As fate would have it, the tiny piece of bone landed directly in the middle of a lower molar on the left side of my mouth. With one quick chewing motion, the upper opposing molar pushed that bone further into the lower molar and split it open, just like a perfectly split diamond that received just the right tap in just the right spot. The pain was immediate, as was the realization that an immediate dental appointment was mandatory.

When I finally saw the dentist, a friend of mine who whom I occasionally played racquetball, he quickly examined the tooth and declared that I needed a "root canal" on the tooth, and that it was best done by a specialist to whom he referred me about 30 minutes north in Lafayette, Louisiana.

The only thought I had at the time was that root canals were always comically associated with excruciating pain and an overall ordeal ("That's about as much fun as a root canal"). So, I looked for reassurance from my friend that it wouldn't be the worst experience of my life, and he patiently explained that this dentist was extremely attentive in the anesthesia department, and that I would have no problems. And he was right. It was a snap. All that worrying for nothing...

The pain was immediate, as was the realization that an immediate dental appointment was mandatory.

Then it was back to life as usual. My tooth always felt fine, and I had absolutely no problems chewing on it. Modern dentistry, it appeared to me, had done its job just fine. I had experienced a problem, and now it was definitively resolved. If only that had been true—but maybe it was good that it wasn't true, since it lead to incredible and profound changes in my life down the road. At least in my own life, some of the most important positive changes and new directions that I have experienced have resulted directly from enormously negative events pushing me in directions that I would never have otherwise chosen. But it would take a while longer, about 5 years longer, for me to be "pushed" into the next major change in my life. For those readers who believe we all have a destiny to fulfill, this probably makes a lot of sense. In retrospect, everything now makes enormous sense, although I did not have a hint of that perspective at the time.

Dream Move Interrupted by a Hard Shove Onto a New Path

For a number of personal reasons, I felt my time as a cardiologist in New Iberia had run its course by 1991, and I decided to move to Colorado Springs, Colorado to continue my professional career. I had always loved Colorado in my many skiing trips there, I was still single and I would not be disrupting anyone's life but my own with a major move, and I decided it was the next significant step and direction for my life, from both an emotional and a logical point of view.

Colorado Springs did not turn out to be the pot of gold at the end of the rainbow for me. I never really enjoyed my life there anywhere close to the level of enjoyment that I had in New Iberia. As it turned out, another major negative event was ultimately awaiting me to push me into a whole new life direction.

After a few years, I had built up a significant solo practice in cardiology, particularly at one of the two hospitals I worked at in the city. It soon became apparent to me that my success was making a number of other cardiologists less than pleased. I had absolutely no "power" at this hospital. However, the hospital was very interested in making the

5-member cardiology group happy, as the income generated by them, including all the cardiac procedures and the many heart surgeries that resulted, was enormous. Had they ever taken most or all of their business to the other hospital in town, this hospital would have had enormous financial difficulty. Paranoid-sounding or not, they were looking to drive me out. Ultimately, they succeeded, although it ended up being on my terms.

I received a notice to appear before a hospital committee to review the "quality" of my work and to determine whether I should be allowed to keep my privileges.

I received a notice to appear before a hospital committee to review the "quality" of my work and to determine whether I should be allowed to keep my privileges. Several, perhaps all, of the cardiologists in the group of 5 made formal assertions that my complication rate was too high in my angiograms and angioplasties. Fortunately, I was able to determine the specifics of these charges before the committee finally met.

I hired a lawyer, but she never made it from Denver to Colorado Springs in time for the meeting, and she was of little to no help in the presentation I assembled. Perhaps the legal education I was to later receive began emerging before I ever went to law school, I don't know.

Armed with the knowledge of the charges, along with knowledge that there was no factual basis for those charges, I put together a 25-page explanation of the nature of the coronary artery angioplasty procedure, along with the pathological and anatomic damage it is known to cause in the selective tearing it inflicts on the arterial wall. I supported all of this information with multiple citations in the current medical literature. Additionally, I clearly demonstrated that my "complication"

> *I clearly demonstrated that my "complication" rate was not only **not** increased, it was substantially lower.*

rate was not only **not** increased, it was substantially lower than the typical complication rate reported in the medical literature of the day. I still had no assurance that these facts would win the day, as one of the group of 5 cardiologists, I had heard, had gone so far as to call me a "butcher" in the cardiac cath lab to members of the committee. Not surprisingly and more than ironically, he was the true butcher, as I had never seen a cardiologist perform procedures in a cath lab with such reckless abandon and lack of attention to multiple important details. But the committee was addressing me, not him, and an energetic exchange of "He said, she said" was going to do me no good at all.

The committee was large, as I seem to remember roughly 20 to 30 doctors and other hospital staff in attendance. I handed copies of my explanation and analysis to all of them, and I then proceeded to read the entire document out loud as they each followed with their individual copy.

Following a very few questions after the reading of the document, I was asked to wait outside. Shortly thereafter, I was informed that there would be no curtailment of my

> *Following a very few questions after the reading of the document, I was asked to wait outside.*

privileges, but that I would need a "monitor"—one of the group of 5—for my cardiac procedures for a while going forward. I must say, I was stunned that my privileges were not taken away; it had seemed like a kangaroo court all the way. However, it appeared my written explanation saved the day. My only friend on the committee later told me, "You really blew them away with your analysis and references to the literature. I guess you just can't push around a Johns Hopkins/Tulane doc without the science on your side." I didn't know if all that was completely true, but it was good to hear.

I immediately decided that I would wait a month, resign my privileges at the hospital, and do all my work at the other hospital. I knew that with future hospital privilege and malpractice insurance applications, the sudden quitting after a hospital inquiry would always raise a red flag. However, I had to go, as the literal wave of nausea that hit me every time I passed through the hospital entrance was too much to deal with on a regular basis.

However, there was still one big problem, or at least it seemed so at the time. The moment I terminated my privileges at this hospital, my income, and my workload, would be pretty much cut in half. There were many patients in Colorado Springs who would only go to one hospital and never the other. However, this did not deter me in following through with the decision to leave.

A few months later, while staring at the walls of my office in my now very low-volume practice, I began to wonder where I was going and the significance of what I was doing.

A few months later, while staring at the walls of my office in my now very low-volume practice, I began to wonder where I was going and the significance of what I was doing. I still enjoyed my cardiology practice, and I felt that I was really helping my patients, but it just didn't seem like it was **enough**. I had no idea what I should be doing as well or instead, but I just had an overwhelming feeling that practicing regular "mainstream" cardiology was not what I wanted to be doing the rest of my life, or that it was part of my true life's path. Instead, it felt like a bridge to something else. But where did the bridge lead?

Medicine that Truly Makes Patients Well—Taught by a Dentist!

Then, a few months later still, I met Dr. Hal Huggins at an alternative energy conference in town. We chatted, had lunch, and he was very insistent that I visit him and check out his dental clinic in town. I certainly had the time and it seemed interesting, so I took him up on his offer shortly thereafter.

Dr. Huggins' clinic was nothing short of amazing. I saw patients clinically improving and abnormal laboratory tests normalizing with a program of dental revision, diet, supplementation, and lifestyle changes to a degree that I had never seen and that I did not believe was possible regardless of the treatment given. My second, and certainly my most significant, medical education was about to begin. And a dentist was going to turn out to be my most significant medical teacher.

Dr. Huggins asked me to start doing consultative work on the many patients that came through the clinic, especially in their follow-up evaluations in the weeks and months after their typically two-week visit to his clinic. He offered a gen-

> *I saw patients clinically improving and abnormal laboratory tests normalizing... to a degree that I had never seen and that I did not believe was possible.*

erous compensation for this work, and I was more than happy to take him up on his offer.

Things started going so well that I began to question the relevancy of my small, ongoing cardiology practice. I was learning an enormous amount of information on toxins, nutrition, and antioxidants like vitamin C. It was all information that had never been addressed at any level of my medical education in the past. Also, Dr. Huggins gave frequent conferences for dentists and physicians from around the world, and I began lecturing regularly with him.

> *I was learning an enormous amount of information on toxins, nutrition, and antioxidants like vitamin C. It was all information that has never been addressed at any level of my medical education in the past.*

I finally terminated my cardiology practice about a year after I met Dr. Huggins, and I have never looked back. I have also not regretted it to even the slightest degree. I just thank God that I was given the opportunity to take that new direction in my professional life. And I had the group of 5 to thank! It certainly never would have happened without them. They gave me the time to think and the ability to take advantage of my first meeting with Dr. Huggins. I am absolutely certain that I would not have abandoned a full-time cardiology practice to explore a new direction with Dr. Huggins, but the group of 5 gave me a possibility that would never have been realized otherwise. From bad came good, once again.

"Only If You Want to Get Well"

Shortly after I signed on "full-time" with my consulting and lecturing with Dr. Huggins, I began to have severe headaches for the first time in my life. I was distressed, to say the least. I finally checked my blood pressure and found that it was very elevated. As a cardiologist, treating high blood pressure in many patients on a regular basis had been my "bread-and-butter," but I never thought I would be dealing with it myself.

I started treating myself with little good clinical response, and I decided to talk to Dr. Huggins, as I still had a small number of mercury fillings in my mouth. Maybe they were the problem. Couldn't hurt to ask.

Huggins cut to the chase: "Do you have any root canals?"

"Well, yes, one. Why?" I replied.

Huggins continued, "You won't get rid of the high blood pressure until you get rid of the root canal."

I was stunned, "That tooth feels fine. You mean I have to get that tooth taken out?"

Huggins didn't miss a beat, "Only if you want to get well." Dr. Huggins' sarcasm was never very endearing, but it was predictable, as I got to know him better.

I already had the highest respect for Dr. Huggins at that point, and I was already enormously frustrated in my attempts to control my blood pressure. I just wanted to trust him (a natural patient sentiment that unfortunately is all too often misplaced), and proceed. The next day the tooth was extracted, and the socket was properly cleaned out. Shortly thereafter, my blood pressure began to normalize, and the headaches completely disappeared. I was stunned, but enormously appreciative at having substantially lowered my chances for eventually getting the stroke or the heart attack that often results from poorly-controlled high blood pressure. I also realized that I needed to learn a *lot* more (like everything) about root canal-treated teeth and their effects throughout the body.

My health actually improved so much that, in retrospect, I had no realization how significantly my health had already deteriorated by the ripe old age of 44. My energy, which I had never considered to be depleted, literally skyrocketed. And my mind also felt "born again" to me, as my concentration and memory improved to a degree I not experienced since beginning medical school roughly 20 years earlier. I pored through books and articles like I never had before.

The improvement of my medical and physical health, along with an excellent income without tremendous demands on my time, led me to my next step: law school.

To this day, I am still not sure why I went, except to say that it felt like the next step in my life. Witnessing the all-too-often travails that Dr. Huggins endured legally played a role in my decision as well, I am quite sure.

Dr. Huggins was never shy or timid in promoting the scientific models that he developed in treating dental conditions and improving medical diseases. And while many dentists and physicians worshiped the ground he walked on for the differences he was making in the lives of so many patients, many more dentists and physicians reviled him just as intensely, and they went out of their way to legally disrupt him in any manner that they could. Dr. Huggins actually had a lawyer on retainer to deal with the literal stream of negative events that eventuated from his dental and educational activities.

The next day the tooth was extracted... My health actually improved so much that, in retrospect, I had no realization how significantly my health had already deteriorated.

Although I have never practiced a single day of law in my life since receiving my law degree and then passing the bar in 1999, I feel the effort was worth it. Medicine, along with everything else we experience in our daily lives, has an enormous amount of legally-based issues that regulate and affect **how** it is practiced, along with what is **allowed** to be practiced.

There is no area of our lives in the United States where we have less freedom today than in the type of medical therapies we get to choose for ourselves. While our medical freedoms have slowly expanded since the Internet, the smartphone, and the dawn of an exciting new Information Age from which nobody can completely insulate themselves, we are still very far from being free of the overreach in healthcare extended by the government and the medical and dental organizations to which they largely give free reign in their treatment of the public. And this is compounded by a legal system that typically goes with the "majority rules" mindset in ruling on critical medical issues, even though significant progress often comes from those in the avant-garde minority. In science and medicine, when the majority rules in the place of scientific data and clear-cut results, everyone loses, except Big Pharma and their dedicated foot soldiers.

In science and medicine, when the majority rules in the place of scientific data and clear-cut results, everyone loses, except Big Pharma and their dedicated foot soldiers.

Shortly after I received my law degree, I published my first book, *Uninformed Consent: The*

Hidden Dangers in Dental Care as a coauthor with Dr. Huggins. Since then, 8 more books and booklets have followed. What has amazed me a bit in retrospect is how all of the books have meshed together in the messages they deliver. It was certainly not completely intentional at the outset, yet they all very much lay down the scientific foundations for the concept of all diseases being caused and promoted by toxins and increased oxidative stress, along with the only truly effective therapies being those that can result in a build-up of antioxidant stores at the cellular level.

Friend's Ailing Heart Demonstrates the Danger of Root Canal-Treated Teeth

About 10 years ago now, I witnessed what was, at the time, another life-altering event for me, at least in terms of how it shaped my thinking, especially with regard to the internal medicine subspeciality that I had chosen, studied, and practiced for so many years: cardiology.

I had just become a consultant to LivOn Laboratories, the producers of liposome-encapsulated nutrients, particularly vitamin C, when the owner of the company began to relate his own personal experience to me about the struggles he was experiencing with coronary artery disease. First diagnosed with heart disease only four years earlier, he described to me a clinical story that revealed what I could only describe as an incredibly aggressive, rapidly evolving type of atherosclerosis in his coronary arteries. In this fairly short period of time he had already experienced seven angioplasties and stent placements, always with a good technical result, yet his coronary artery disease continue to rage in the rest of his arteries.

I already knew about the effects of root canal-treated teeth on heart disease and heart attacks, although I had not yet done much of the research I was yet to do on this subject before publishing my book, *Stop America's #1 Killer! Reversible Vitamin Deficiency Found to be Origin of ALL Coronary Heart Disease*. Nevertheless, I was already convinced that having root canal-treated teeth was a significant risk factor in the development of coronary atherosclerosis and eventual heart attack.

My friend called me one day, more than a bit depressed, and began relating how much new angina pain he was experiencing. His depression was more than understandable, since his numerous angioplasties did not seem to give him any long-term clinical stability whatsoever. Furthermore, without any exaggeration, the supplement regimen he was following was truly amazing. I had never, before or since, encountered anyone who was taking such a highly-dosed and wide array of **quality** nutrient supplements. I was amazed that he had any room left in his stomach to eat. He was even taking about nine grams of liposome-encapsulated vitamin C at that time, an amount that I have since found to resolve almost every clinical circumstance in which it was used.

He was in Las Vegas. I was in Denver, having relocated from Colorado Springs after finishing law school. I immediately advised him to fly over to me, and that I would take him the following morning to my personal dentist who I knew would do correctly and thoroughly whatever needed to be done. My friend had no idea whether he had one or more root canal-treated teeth in his mouth, but I felt certain there had to be at least one.

> *He had already experienced seven angioplasties and stent placements, always with a good technical result, yet his coronary artery disease continued to rage in the rest of his arteries.*

He arrived, we had a bite to eat, and he went to his hotel room for the evening. When I arrived to pick him up the next morning, he was sitting in the lobby, appearing very depressed and even a bit teary-eyed as he related to me how much chest pain he had experienced throughout the night. He indicated that he saw no point any longer in going to see the dentist. I told him that was **not** an option, and I managed to get him into my car.

My dentist found only **ONE** root canal-treated tooth, and he promptly extracted it and cleaned out the infected bone remaining in the socket.

As amazing as this might sound to many people, my friend never had a single angina pain again. Furthermore, he had the opportunity to have a cardiac CT scan with venous contrast several years later (he was having no symptoms), and much of his arterial narrowing documented on earlier angiograms had resolved. In other words, after the one root canal-treated tooth came out, he stopped having chest pain, he stopped evolving further coronary artery narrowings, and he largely **reversed** the critical narrowings that had been seen earlier. For me, it was a combined scientific and emotional experience that remains hard to define.

> *A cardiac CT scan with venous contrast several years later... [showed that] much of his arterial narrowing documented on earlier angiograms had resolved.*

This experience with my friend's heart disease and its positive response to the extraction of his only root canal-treated tooth directly led me to plunge into the substantial research cited in my next book at that time, *Stop America's #1 Killer!* The research involved in writing this book taught me an enormous amount about cardiology, a disease that I already felt held no significant secrets from me. I couldn't have been more wrong. My training had taught me what to do after unstable angina or a heart attack had presented. I humbly realized as I combed through the literature that I had known, like most of my fellow cardiologists, very little as to why heart disease developed in the first place, and why some people can do everything right and still develop a problem with coronary atherosclerosis.

It was the research for this book, along with the writing and researching of the next book, *Primal Panacea*, that finally caused me to realize that all diseases are secondary to increased oxidative stress in the affected cells and tissues. It also became apparent to me that focal infections, such as seen in root canal-treated

I humbly realized as I combed through the literature that I had known, like most of my fellow cardiologists, very little as to why heart disease developed in the first place.

teeth, infected gums, and other infected teeth, reliably promoted increased oxidative stress via the dissemination of pathogens and pathogen-generated toxins throughout the body. Wherever the pathogens and toxins ended up and/or concentrated most would determine the degree of increased oxidative stress and ultimately the disease process that an individual would demonstrate. This all coalesced into the realization as to why the presence of root canal-treated teeth was a major risk factor for heart disease. This was because the steady stream of pathogens and toxins released from such teeth first encountered the high-pressure arterial system in the coronary arteries. Upon getting seeded there, the pathogens rapidly consume all the vitamin C present, and the focal scurvy that is initiated causes a chronic inflammatory response, which never resolves until the focal infection source is removed.

The Negative Health Impact of an Oral Focal Infection Hits Home Again

Focal infection again hit home for me personally about two and a half years ago. I had basically good baseline health, but the laboratory testing that I had been following for years continued to show significant elevations in the CRP (C-reactive protein) levels, which is a strong indicator of chronic inflammation somewhere in the body, and it is also a significant risk factor for coronary heart disease and heart attack. I had been disturbed by its elevation, but I could not figure out how to get it down and resolve whatever the inflammatory/infective focus was in my body that might be causing it. However, I was convinced that I would eventually become another heart attack patient if I could not resolve it. I had even taken 100 grams of vitamin C intravenously daily for a week at one point, rechecked the test, and found that I only knocked it down a little bit, and only for a fairly brief time.

Then, on May 30, 2012, I chased a hostile neighborhood dog away from attacking my toy poodle. I was almost immediately stopped in my tracks with a sudden shortness of breath and tightness in my chest. I slowly and carefully walked back into my house and sat down. Within about 5 minutes, the symptoms had all resolved. I then recalled that I probably had similar symptoms a few months earlier when walking uphill, but I had pretty much gone into denial and decided to pay it no attention. However, I was a cardiologist. I had seen similar scenarios untold number of times in my own patients. There was no denying or dismissing this episode.

I was almost immediately stopped in my tracks with a sudden shortness of breath and tightness in my chest.

To me, the conclusion was inescapable. I now had a critical or sub-critical narrowing in one or more coronary arteries, and the encounter with the hostile dog had almost pushed me to a heart attack. I took very large amounts of IV vitamin C (100 or more grams daily) and many grams of liposome-encapsulated vitamin C orally for the next week. I also arranged to have a tonsillectomy at the end of that week.

A tonsillectomy? Dr. Josef Issels wrote on his experiences with treating advanced cancer patients back in the 1940s and 1950s. He noted that 97% of them had root canal-treated or otherwise infected teeth, and his treatment protocol, which was highly effective in resolving cancer and increasing longevity, began in the dental chair with the extraction of those teeth. He also routinely had these patients undergo tonsillectomy, even when the tonsils appeared grossly normal, and there had been no known occurrences of tonsillar infection by history. And perhaps most interestingly, nearly all the extracted tonsils showed evidence of significant ongoing infections and abscesses, even those that had appeared normal by routine examination.

I had always reasoned that the presence of root canal-treated teeth suffused the tonsils... with an overwhelmingly large pathogen and toxin exposure.

Because of the experiences reported by Dr. Issels, I had always reasoned that the presence of root canal-treated teeth suffused the tonsils, especially the one on the side of the root canal-treated teeth, with an overwhelmingly large pathogen and toxin exposure. Many tonsils in younger people needed extraction because they were unable to completely return to normal after one or more bouts of tonsillitis. It appeared that the capacity of the tonsil to deal with an orally-based infection was significantly limited, and the "24/7" exposure to a root canal-treated tooth quite rapidly overwhelmed this capacity. In fact, largely based on Dr. Issels' findings, it appeared to me that the root canal-treated tooth could be relied upon to convert an otherwise normal tonsil from **protector** to **infector** in fairly short order. How long did the root canal-treated tooth need to trash the tonsil? Hard to say. A month, a year? Probably no more than that.

Since I was at the end of my clinical rope, I called an ENT doctor. I absolutely lied through my teeth and told him that I was sick and tired of having tonsillitis so many times in the last few years, and that since the tonsils were "settled down now" and in between infections, now would be a great time to take them out. He agreed, as I had earlier looked up the "indications" for tonsillectomy in an adult, and I made sure my "history" filled all the clinical requirements needed by the surgeon to proceed with the procedure.

Before the surgery, the ENT doc commented that my tonsils looked completely normal, but were perhaps a little enlarged. After the surgery was completed and I was fully recovered from the anesthesia, he came by to do a quick post-op look. He commented that everything looked fine. I asked him if he had noticed anything else of interest when he did the surgery. He replied:

"Well, now that you mention it, when I grabbed the left tonsil to begin taking it out, I caused a bunch of pus to starting coming out. It was pretty impressive."

Two things should be noted here. The left side was the side where my root canal-treated tooth had been, even though it had been extracted about 18 years earlier. The second thing to note is that I had never had any form of tonsillitis in my life. It appeared very clear to me that root canals can trash tonsils, and that once-trashed, the affected tonsil(s) stayed trashed. My left tonsil had 18 years to recover and resume normal function, supported by a very good diet and great supplementation, and it could not do it.

However, let me also hasten to add that I would never advise an adult to get a tonsillectomy unless the indications were clear that it was needed to improve health after all other reasonable interventions had failed in reaching that goal. While I could not have been happier to have my tonsils out, especially after learning they were filled with pus, I have never had a worse experience in my life. Being a bit too macho for my own good, I went directly into my post-operative period without any help from anyone. In fact, I was continuing to care for my 90-year-old mother at the same time I was trying to recover my own health.

While I knew that tonsillectomies were a much bigger deal for adults than kids, I had no idea how much different the experience would be. At least for me, the post-operative phase was pure torture, and remained so for at least a full month. It took that long to reasonably start swallowing small portions of a regular diet. For the first week just swallowing water was inconceivably difficult. Because of this, my overall state of dehydration was exaggerated to the point that I would wake up in the middle of the night with the mucous membranes in my mouth and throat literally stuck to each other, in need of significant effort to get them separated again. It was the most peculiar and perhaps the most unpleasant sensation I have ever endured.

On the fifth post-operative night I woke up in the middle of the night and realized that I had been having bizarre dreams and even some hallucinations upon awakening, and that I was losing my general orientation. Somehow, in the middle of this altered mental state, I still was able to appreciate that I had not urinated for almost an entire day. For someone who typically drinks at least 2 to 3 quarts of water daily and urinates at least 8 times daily, I knew things were not going well for my body. I wanted badly to just go back to sleep, but I was quite afraid that in my advanced state of fluid depletion that I might not wake up again. Instead, I forced myself to prepare an IV of vitamin C and sterile water and administer it to myself. A couple hours later I urinated a bit, and I followed that with two more infusions over the next 4 to 5 hours. I was still miserable, but the urine was flowing once again, and at least I now felt I would survive.

In spite of this experience, I knew the tonsillectomy was necessary for my survival, or perhaps more accurately, to avoid the progression of my

> *I would wake up in the middle of the night with the mucous membranes in my mouth and throat literally stuck to each other.*

chest pain to the point of a heart attack. My general health improved rapidly after the surgery (and the prolonged, problematic post-operative period), and my laboratory tests improved as well. But they did not normalize. The CRP remained elevated, but substantially less so.

In spite of this experience, I knew the tonsillectomy was necessary for my survival, or perhaps more accurately, to avoid the progression of my chest pain to the point of a heart attack.

Roughly 6 months later, I had an opportunity to get a rapid cardiac CAT scan with injection of venous contrast. This allowed me for the first time in my life to visualize my coronary arteries. Sure enough, in the middle of the left anterior descending coronary artery, which is the most important heart artery in most people, there was a 40 to 50% narrowed area. I suspected that this area of narrowing had been critical, probably 70% or more, six months earlier. I knew, however, that when the bulk of infectious toxicity is removed from the body and high enough doses of antioxidants are taken on a regular basis, atherosclerosis will typically regress and sometimes revert to even an angiographically normal status. My coronary artery calcium score was zero at the time of the cardiac CAT scan, which further indicated to me that my overall diet, lifestyle, and supplementation regimen was pretty good, as long as I could avoid focal infections such as my root canal-treated tooth and the secondary chronically infected tonsil(s).

Around the beginning of 2013, I discovered that I was low in thyroid function and very low in my testosterone levels. Once again, my own medical problems led me to research and eventually write about the importance of sex hormones and thyroid function, which I had never really addressed before. These two issues ended up being discussed extensively in my latest book, *Death by Calcium: Proof of the toxic effects of dairy and calcium supplementation.*

I began taking dessicated thyroid hormone on a daily basis. Also, twice weekly I began intramuscular testosterone injections. Once again, after a few months of this new therapy, my health "jumped" another level in terms of energy and the need for only 7 to 8 hours of sleep nightly rather than 10. It once again brought home to me how good health can slowly but surely decline over the years, along with how very difficult it is to realize at any given point in time how significant this loss has been.

I was reasonably satisfied that I had done everything of importance in eliminating focal infection(s) from my body. However, my CRP still had not dropped into the normal range yet, and I kept on wondering what I was missing.

Another Dental Event Confirms the Danger of Infected Teeth

In January of 2014, I had another dental "event." I was giving several lectures on vitamin C in Algeria, and my upper left second molar began to hurt. This had been a tooth that had been heavily decayed in the past and had undergone numerous filling procedures before finally being crowned about six months earlier. I took antibiotics and ibuprofen and hoped for the best. I was dreading having a crescendo of pain in the plane trip back across the Atlantic.

Very fortunately, the tooth settled down, and the pain disappeared completely after about a week. I saw a dentist locally in Biloxi, where I had lived for the last five years caring for my mother, and X-rays showed no obvious sign of infection. I chewed normally on the tooth for another five months.

The tooth then began to just not feel "right." It was not painful, and I could usually chew anything I wanted on it. However, I knew something was amiss. At times it did hurt just a little when I chewed, and I knew that was never normal and certainly not a good sign for long-term tooth health. My CRP was still not normal, and my body/health intuition told me once again that there was still another focal infection to be addressed.

After ruminating on all of this for another month, and after reliving in my mind all that I had already gone through to reclaim my health and avoid having a heart attack, I decided that the tooth had to be extracted. I can't say that I would ever be completely comfortable advising a patient to have such a tooth extracted with such little clear evidence of infection or pathology being present. However, this was my body, my tooth, and my health. I wanted it out, and if it turned out to be a completely normal tooth, then it was still completely on me and nobody else. I flew to my dentist in Denver to have the procedure done.

At times it did hurt just a little when I chewed, and I knew that was never normal and certainly not a good sign for long-term tooth health.

I had the X-ray taken again, and this time there was the suggestion of possible infection. Mind you, I was still going to have the tooth extracted even if the X-ray had been completely normal. I wasn't sure if this was a better quality X-ray than I had six months earlier or whether the X-ray finding was truly new.

When the tooth came out, there were abscesses on each root tip, and there was further abscess and infection in the socket. All of this was meticulously debrided and cleaned out, along with complete removal of the periodontal ligament in order to optimize healing and the filling-in of new bone. I suspect that the extensive decay in this tooth many years earlier had progressed to a long-standing low grade chronic pulpal infection that recently became more acute.

Roughly two months later (late July 2014) I had my CRP retested. To my great satisfaction, the result was 2.02. The normal range for LabCorp on this test is 0.00 to 3.00. This test had been checked seven different times during the past one and one-half years. The average of those seven tests was 4.94, a very high and very abnormal CRP, almost certainly reflecting significant chronic inflammation in my body. But the infected tooth was now gone, and the CRP was well within the range of normal. For me, the concept of focal infection and its effects throughout the body is now a simple fact, as the removal of the infected tooth clearly normalized my CRP level. Chronic inflammation always accompanies coronary heart disease, and for the moment I am now comfortable that my risk for a heart attack has been significantly reduced.

CHAPTER NINE

ALTERNATIVES *to Root Canal Treatment*

Some Healthy Options

Several options exist to help out the patient who has had one or more root canal-treated teeth extracted, or to the patient who just elects to get an infected tooth extracted first before even proceeding to a root canal treatment. These options include bridges, partials or full dentures depending on the remaining mouth anatomy, implants, and doing nothing. Doing nothing is not a good option in many circumstances, but it can sometimes be the best option when the back molar is missing but chewing is not compromised.

It goes without saying that a healthy mouth that is free of cavities and free of periodontal disease is ideal. However, even with the most diligent home care regimen, tooth decay can sometimes occur which may eventually lead to pulp infection.

In addition, damage to teeth caused by trauma can be the indication for a root canal procedure or tooth extraction. The question, then, is: What are the restoration options when the tooth pulp becomes infected, and the tooth is extracted rather than given a root canal procedure?

When the infected tooth needs to be extracted, the restoration options include:

1) Leaving the space empty

2) Restoring the missing tooth or empty space(s) with a removable partial denture (RPD)

3) Restoring the empty space(s) with a permanently cemented fixed bridge

4) Restoring the space(s) with dental implant(s)

However, because the ADA has unequivocally stated that root canal-treated teeth are 100% safe and can pose no systemic health risks whatsoever, patients will likely be led towards having a root canal procedure instead of an RPD, fixed bridge, or dental implant. Considering the ADA's position on the root canal procedure, the encouragement to go in this direction is completely understandable.

To further complicate matters, if a patient decides to have a fixed bridge and somewhere down the line one of the abutment (anchoring) teeth becomes non-vital, the patient will have to make the choice to have a root canal procedure on that abutment tooth or to have that tooth extracted which necessitates removal of the entire bridge. After paying a sizable price for the fixed bridge, many people would be reluctant to remove the entire bridge that could have been "saved" with just a root canal procedure. Now the patient faces additional expense for a new bridge or dental implants. So the treatment decision is definitely not an easy one for the patient, especially when considering all of the expenses involved.

The decision to have a root canal procedure should be made by the individual patient who has been completely informed about all of the risks and benefits of the procedure.

As all root canal-treated teeth remain infected, the ability to tolerate a root canal-treated tooth varies widely from individual to individual, as does the degree of tooth toxicity. Extensive work by Dr. Boyd Haley did not find a single extracted root canal-treated tooth that did not have significant toxicity. And Dr. Haley tested over 5,000 consecutive extracted root canal-treated teeth. How these toxins will impact the health of any given individuals could vary greatly based on some known factors—such as genetic predispositions, immune status, antioxidant status, age, and general health—as well as by a future health status that cannot be known. Therefore, the final treatment decision should always rest with the completely informed patient.

Now let's address in more detail the treatment options to restore the empty space after extraction.

"Do Nothing" Option

The first option is to do nothing. This may be an acceptable permanent option if the tooth that was extracted is a second molar. Most of the chewing is done from the first molar forward so it is very unlikely, functionally speaking, that this tooth would ever be missed. The only downside of leaving the second molar space vacant is the continued eruption of the opposing tooth. If there is no opposing tooth, or if there is partial occlusion of the opposing tooth by the first molar, then continued eruption of the opposing tooth will not occur.

Removable Partial Denture Option

If the extracted tooth is any other tooth besides the second molar or a wisdom tooth, then the empty space should be restored both for aesthetic reasons and, more importantly, to maintain the stability of the dental arch and the ability to chew optimally. The least invasive restoration to replace missing teeth is a removable partial denture (RPD). A RPD rests on the gum tissue and hooks onto the remaining teeth with various types of clasps. A RPD is completely removable so it is easily taken out of the mouth to clean.

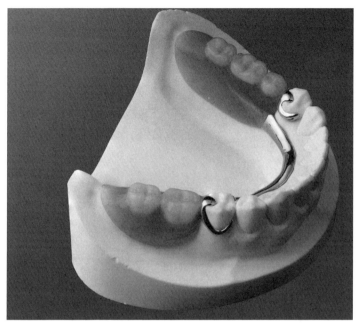

Figure 9-1: A partial denture as a replacement for 5 lower molars. This appliance is removable for cleaning.

Fixed Bridge Option

Another option to replace missing teeth is a fixed bridge. A fixed bridge uses the teeth (called abutment teeth) on either side of the empty space as supports for crowns to fill in the space. The abutment teeth are prepared for crowns in the same way as for a regular crown procedure. Then, a one-piece restoration is fabricated where a tooth or teeth that are to fill in the empty space are connected to the two abutment crowns and the entire unit is fitted and cemented permanently in place. The major downside of this procedure is that a lot of natu-

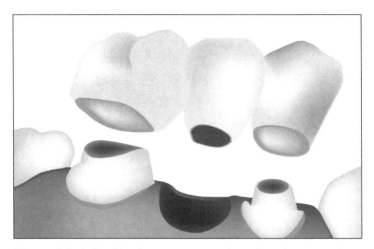

Figure 9-2: A fixed bridge is permanently anchored to a tooth on either side. The anchor teeth must be filed down to accomodate the caps that hold the replacement tooth.

ral tooth structure must be removed in the crown abutment preparation, which can sometimes lead to death of the pulp tissue. If both of the abutment teeth already have very large dental restorations in them, then only slightly more natural tooth preparation will be necessary and this option becomes more attractive.

Dental Implant Option

Dental implants have become a very predictable and reliable long-term solution to replacing a missing tooth. This procedure involves the implantation of a sterile titanium post as an abutment in the extraction site. The implant serves the same supporting function as the natural tooth or the root

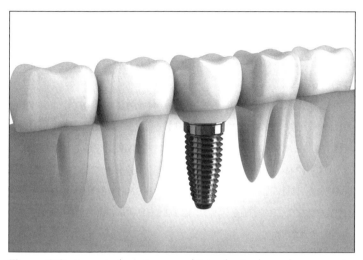

Figure 9-3: A surgical post screwed into the jawbone becomes the anchor for the replacement tooth in a dental implant.

canal-treated tooth prepared as the support for a single crown or fixed bridge without the negative health impact delivered by bacteria and toxins leaking out of the root canal-treated tooth.

When placed in healthy, well-healed bone a dental implant can provide many years of function without the need to place crowns on teeth adjacent to the empty space in order to place a fixed bridge. Depending on the particular situation, an implant can be used to replace a single tooth or as an abutment for a bridge.

When performed as outlined below, a dental implant is always preferable to a root canal-treated tooth because a root canal-treated tooth can always be expected to negatively impact health substantially more than an implant, especially if it was properly-placed. Indeed, a properly-placed implant should have no discernible negative impact on general health.

Although some dental implants are placed immediately after extraction and are sometimes immediately restored, it is recommended that a dental implant procedure should not be started until new healthy bone has filled the extraction site. This important healing process requires a minimum of three months.

Unless bone grafts or sinus augmentation is needed to create more bone volume, the implant procedure is a painless and relatively straightforward procedure for a dentist trained in implant dentistry. Once the bone at the implant site is carefully measured, both by physical exam and X-ray evaluation, the dentist will select the appropriate implant size. An incision is made in the gum tissue to expose the top of the bone. Then a series of increasing diameter drills create a hole in the jawbone, and a sterile post made of titanium alloy is firmly screwed into place. When the top of the implant is flush with the bone crest, the gum tissue is sutured closed. The implant remains untouched under the gum tissue for three to six months as the bone heals and matures and essentially locks the implant into place.

After sufficient healing time the restorative process begins by reopening the gum tissue and an implant abutment is inserted onto the exposed implant. This implant abutment acts the same way as a natural tooth that has been prepared for a crown. At this point the restoration proceeds essentially the same way in which a crown is placed on a prepared natural tooth.

It is very important that the gum tissue around the implant be kept very clean, as the gum tissue does not insert fibers into the implant abutment like a natural tooth does to prevent bacteria from reaching the underlying bone. However, if this gum tissue is kept clean and plaque-free, it will keep a firm seal around the implant abutment, and it is likely that no bacteria will migrate into the bone.

The goal of this book is not to eliminate the root canal procedure *per se*. The goal is to state scientific research, to interpret it logically, to stimulate further objective and unbiased research into the safety of root canal-treated teeth, and to allow dental patients to make their own best treatment decisions.

CHAPTER TEN

CONSENTING *to Root Canal Treatment*

Dentistry —
The Right Way

Patients need to understand proposed procedures and treatment protocols as completely as possible in order to make informed medical and dental decisions. At the same time, healthcare providers cannot really overdo their attempts to ensure that a patient fully understands a planned procedure along with the expected benefits and potential negative outcomes and long-term side effects. A healthcare provider's full disclosure and patient agreement prior to treatment is called informed consent. It is the process in which healthcare practitioners and their patients "engage in a dialogue to explain and comprehend the nature, alternatives, and risks of a procedure" or treatment protocol. [1]

This means that a medical or a dental procedure, or a treatment plan, needs to be preceded by:

1. A clear explanation of the procedure, surgery, or planned treatment.

2. Evidence of comprehension of the explanation by the patient, as would be apparent in a meaningful dialogue between caregiver and patient. Comprehension by family members is also important and especially important when there is a possibility of cognitive impairment on the part of the patient.

3. A complete explanation of any possible risks associated with the procedure, surgery, or planned treatment, along with a balanced, scientific analysis of anticipated benefits. This includes a full enumeration of known complications that can occur with a reasonable approximation of the likelihood of their occurrence, including the worst possible outcomes. A reasonable approximation of the likelihood of realizing the therapeutic goal of the procedure, surgery, or planned treatment should also be included. This requires that the healthcare practitioner have an awareness of the pertinent current scientific literature addressing a given procedure, surgery, or planned treatment.

4. A complete explanation of the alternative approaches or options available for the procedure, surgery, or planned treatment.

5. A complete and comprehensive response to any questions that the patient might

pose regarding the procedure, surgery, or planned treatment.

6. Documentation in writing, and preferably by audio/video recording, of the execution of the above informed consent principles.

Many informed consents do not meet the standards outlined above. However, a great deal of legal wrangling and ultimately malpractice suits could be avoided by adhering closely to these standards. Furthermore, the "protection" is equally available for caregiver and patient. Patients need to be protected from inappropriate surgeries and procedures, and healthcare providers also need protection against patients who are litigation-prone, claiming they were never advised of a particular outcome for a given surgery or procedure.

Probably the best mutual protection occurs when everything is recorded. This contains not only precisely what was said and discussed, but also the tones of voice and vocal inflections involved, which are vital in knowing how something was presented or stressed. Such recording might have been problematic or unduly complicated in the past, but the smartphone technology

Patients need to be protected from inappropriate surgeries and procedures, and healthcare providers also need protection against patients who are litigation-prone.

of today makes recording and permanently storing such evidence simple and economically feasible.

Dental Surgeries Are Medical Procedures

While consent forms are routinely filled out for dental surgeries and procedures, these consents typically limit themselves to advising what can happen in the short-term within the mouth only. This is no longer an acceptable form of informed consent. Certainly, many informed consents for medical surgeries and procedures are quite poorly executed as well. The big difference is that a medical patient undergoing any type of surgery is at least presented with a list of the potential adverse outcomes, which nearly always includes the possibility of heart attack in older individuals.

If a patient goes to his dentist with a painful tooth, and a root canal procedure is recommended, the patient must also be made aware of the increased possibility of developing coronary artery disease months or years after the procedure.

The literature has now established this connection, and any dental patient who is not told of this link and who later sustains a heart attack should, in theory, have a *strong dental malpractice suit against the dental practitioner*. But determination of malpractice is based upon the current standard of care. In legal terms, standard of care is the level at which the average, prudent healthcare provider in a given community would practice. So until the dental profession acknowledges these systemic risks, dentists will effectively not be obligated to inform patients of these risks, and patients will still not be making informed decisions. It will likely take several malpractice test cases before the standard of care is sufficiently changed to permit a truly informed consent.

The patient has the absolute right to a complete informed consent as to the dental and medical complications that could potentially result from that procedure.

All dental and medical procedures carry some risk. So once the patient is properly informed of all the risks of a procedure, the dentist has a right to do the procedure, and the patient has the right to receive the procedure. However, the patient has the absolute right to a complete informed consent as to the dental and medical complications that could potentially result from that procedure.

Just like many other procedures in medicine and dentistry, a percentage of root canal-treated teeth will develop recurrent symptoms and have to be re-treated. Patients should be informed of this possibility before deciding to have a root canal procedure performed, as this may be a factor in deciding whether to proceed with the procedure or just to extract the tooth.

Whether Recognized or Not, General Medicine and Dentistry Are Inseparable

Solid research demonstrates the intimate relationship between dental health and overall health. Studies confirm that what happens in the mouth, and specifically in and around the teeth, can have profound implications for the health in the rest of the body. Even so, the evidence showing this connection remains unknown or **actively ignored** by many general dentists, endodontists, and oral surgeons today. It is disturbing that much of the research on the systemic health risks associated with root canal-treated teeth is done in other countries.

Patients should have the right to change their mind at a later date if they decide to extract the tooth after root canal treatment.

It's high time that dentistry is properly encompassed by general medicine. Dentistry is not, and never will be, a profession completely unto itself. Many dental pathologies, infections, and toxins negatively impact the general health of the patient. Denial of these relationships will continue to harm patients and put the long-term viability of a dental practice into increasing legal jeopardy.

The Patient Should Always Have the Right to Choose

Even if the root canal-treated tooth feels perfectly fine, as is often the case, the patient has the right to have it extracted and the dentist has the obligation to extract it when requested. Just as it is the right of the patients to choose either a root canal or an extraction at the time that the tooth pulp first becomes infected, patients should have the right to change their mind at a later date if they decide to extract the tooth after root canal treatment in order to optimally preserve their long-term general health.

Unfortunately, at the time of this writing dentists who are aware of the toxicity of root canal-treated teeth and who are willing to extract them when requested are still in danger of punitive actions against them by their dental boards. When a dentist's action, including the extraction of a root canal-treated tooth, improves the health of a patient, it should be commended. But instead, dentists continue to face disciplinary action for extracting root canal-treated teeth.

The patient who has read this book and no longer wants the toxicity of a root canal-treated tooth circulating in their body needs to **protect** *any dentist willing to extract that tooth.*

Until that changes, the patient who has read this book and no longer wants the toxicity of a root canal-treated tooth circulating in their body needs to **protect** any dentist willing to extract that tooth. Therefore, it is strongly advised that the patient wanting the extraction of a root canal-treated tooth assert two things:

1) The presence of pain in the tooth/jaw
2) The desire not to have a "redo" root canal procedure but to have the tooth extracted

This way, the patient gets what he/she wants (and has the right to), and the dentist is protected by being able to assert in the patient's chart *in writing* that the extraction was warranted due to chronic symptoms along with a specific request not to redo the root canal procedure. Furthermore, the dentist should routinely take a pathological specimen and culture for microorganisms from the base of the extraction site before cleaning out the infection and necrosis and document the presence of those findings with a confirmatory report. Patients and conscientious dentists alike must act in ways to have both their health and their licenses protected.

Patients and conscientious dentists alike must act in ways to have both their health and their licenses protected.

Root Canals and Heart Attacks

While the scientific data being accumulated now clearly show that root canal-treated teeth have at least an equal negative impact on body-wide health as any degree of periodontal disease, that connection can still be regarded medico-legally as "inconclusive" with the absence of direct prospective studies linking the presence of root canal-treated teeth and the incidence/severity of various diseases. However, the connection between the presence of root canal-treated teeth and an increased risk of coronary heart disease is now well-established and scientifically sound.

> Therefore, the individual who has root canal-treated teeth and later has a heart attack or unequivocal evidence of coronary artery disease, such as on coronary angiography, now has a ***sound legal basis*** upon which to sue the dentist who did those procedures and provided no informed consent that such a risk of increased heart disease was at least a possibility.

Unfortunately, unless and until dentists are legally held accountable for the negative health consequences of these procedures, it is unlikely that the truth about root canal-treated teeth will ever properly reach the public awareness. It is our hope that the toxicity of root canal-treated teeth and their involvement in systemic diseases will soon be acknowledged by the dental profession without the need for malpractice lawsuits.

CHAPTER ELEVEN

TESTIMONIALS *about Root Canal Treatment*

Patients Tell Their Stories

The following testimonials represent a small sample of cases where extraction of root canal-treated teeth demonstrated the presence of serious infection and resulted in a dramatic improvement in a variety of systemic conditions. Where appropriate, findings from pathology reports follow the testimonial.

Otherwise Untreatable Headaches

Since an early age, I have had a few root canals on various teeth in the upper left side of my mouth. In early 1999, I started to develop headaches that began on the left temple and radiated to the back of my head, behind my ear and my eye. The pain would come and go and I dealt with it for as long as I could.

I had been seeing my dentist regularly for check-ups and cleanings; in the spring of 1999, I required another root canal in the same spot, the upper left side. During the series of root canal visits, the pain intensified; I was taking four Advil every four hours to alleviate the pain. I could have used something stronger but I could not take narcotics and continue to work as a nurse.

The dentist did try to make an accurate diagnosis of my pain but stated that he felt that it was unrelated to my teeth. I proceeded to have a MRI, a visit with an Ear, Nose, and Throat doctor as well as a full exam with a neurologist. All findings were negative and the headaches remained a mystery.

I returned to my dentist and not being able to make a definitive diagnosis he suggested we pull the tooth that was last root canal treated. It took four weeks to heal because I developed a dry socket. I now was on narcotics, Vicodin to be exact, and still had no relief from headaches. This pain was the worst I have ever experienced; it felt like I had a hole in my gum that was open to the nerves in my face. Ultimately, the gum healed but the headaches persisted. Again, my dentist recommended a pain clinic to me since he could find nothing dentally wrong.

Understanding now that I was at a dead end, I was speaking to my mother-in-law who told me about Dr. Kulacz. She explained that he practiced "integrative dentistry". When I asked her to explain she stated "he takes your whole body into consideration when you have a problem, not just your teeth."

I had nothing to lose; I called Dr. Kulacz in August of 1999. I explained my symptoms to him over the phone; right then and there, he said "it sounds like you have some type of circulation problem to the bone and possible residual infection or dead bone where the extractions were performed. Come and see me right away."

I saw Dr. Kulacz the next day. Within minutes, he had made a definitive diagnosis. "Your pain is from the damage that was caused by use of Novocaine with vasoconstrictors during all of the root canals you have had. In addition, all root canals you had were infected. I would like to remove the affected teeth and infected, dead bone at the extraction sites and your pain will likely be resolved".

I had the surgery a day or two later and my headaches were finally gone. Subsequently, I had a partial bridge placed and have never had the same headache return.

Dr. Kulacz through his knowledge and wisdom truly saved me from a life of pain and potential death from the infection that could have spread to my blood stream. In addition, as a health care provider he has proven that you MUST consider the whole body; not just the teeth.

*Most dentists don't get involved in the
medical history of their patients and most physicians don't get involved with the dental history of their patients. I am so grateful that Dr.
Kulacz took the time to listen to me, analyze
my symptoms, and make the right decisions to
alleviate my pain and let me go on with a normal life. He is truly an incredible dentist and
human being.*

-T.D., R.N., B.S.N., Mahopac, NY

Microscopic pathologic analysis of samples from
the patient above found globules of a gray/translu-
cent foreign material coated by polymorphonuclear
neutrophils (PMNs) and coccal bacterial colonies.
PMNs are a type of phagocyte produced by the
immune system to fight inflammation and infection,
and they are the predominant cells in pus. PMNs
are also seen with lymphocytes in small fragments
of necrotic fibrovascular tissue. The findings were
consistent with subacute osteomyelitis (bone infection) with foreign material and bacterial colonies.
The full pathology report on tissues obtained from
the patient appears in Appendix E.

Chronic Arthritis Relief

Dear Dr. Kulacz:
*There is no way I can thank you enough
for helping me to get back to an active life
again.*

As you know I was wearing a brace on my knee, so I could hold off getting a knee replacement. I did get some relief.

Since you extracted two bottom teeth, which were infected, I have not been wearing my knee brace. I'm able to play golf and walk without discomfort. Overall, my arthritis is about 85% better.

Thank you and God bless,

-M.D., New York

Facial Neuralgia

Dear Dr. Kulacz:

Today marks the beginning of a new lease on life for me. I had a wonderful day thinking about how lucky I am to finally get a second chance to enjoy all those things with which I am so truly blessed. You know my story; but just for the record, I will summarize.

This past January, I decided to bridge my lower left molars: That was the sorriest day of my life. Each and every aspect of my life was compromised from that point on. I endured the most excruciating pain I had every experienced in my entire life which includes a 20-hour labor and delivery. My mouth was numbed repeatedly during endodontic procedures, many times without success. I experienced temporary face paralysis and repeated infections as well as many, many extremely unpleasant procedures—all without relieving any of my pain.

*The only way I was able to make it through
each day was with the help of my very support-
ive friends and family. There were many nights
I did not want to face another day and began
to understand why people end their lives.*

*Short of pulling two teeth out of my
mouth, I was referred to a neurologist who
diagnosed me with facial neuralgia and pre-
scribed Neurontin. The pain was somewhat
relieved but I was unable to function as I am
accustomed due to extreme fatigue and for-
getfulness. The pain did eventually return and
intensify.*

*As a last resort, I chose an alternative
route—acupuncture. Fortunately for me, my
Family Nurse Practitioner and Acupuncturist
had just met you and thought you could possibly help me. After my conversation with you,
I was upset to hear that the teeth I had been
holding onto in vain would have to be removed
and the bone tissue cleaned out properly. At
that point, I was way beyond the "end of my
rope" so I consented to the surgery. All the
information I received from you was truly
remarkable and professional and I had no
doubt you would indeed help me.*

*I wasn't the slightest bit nervous going
into the procedure. The procedure itself was
painless, without incident. You and your anesthesiologist, Dr. Greenspan, were a pleasure*

to deal with, and I will be an advocate in your crusade to educate those who suffer needlessly.

-T.S., New Jersey

Largely Pain Free

Dr. Kulacz performed cavitational surgery in the sites of three of my extracted wisdom teeth on July 12, 2000.

I was referred to Dr. Kulacz by my local dentist in Pennsylvania, because an ultrasound test indicated that I had fairly deep cavitations in my lower jaw on both right and left sides. In addition, one of my friends had recently undergone extensive cavitational surgery by Dr. Kulacz and highly recommended him to me.

Before undergoing surgery, I was given a packet of information including forms to be completed concerning my health history, information about techniques that would be used in my surgery, and pre- and post-surgical protocol. I was glad both to be well informed myself and that Dr. Kulacz would be well informed about my condition before my surgery. This information also assured me that much care would be taken to safeguard my health and to prevent further infection.

On the day of my surgery, my husband and I were given more than adequate time to discuss matters with Dr. Kulacz. Having heard various stories and rumors, I was somewhat concerned about possible nerve damage. Dr. Kulacz, by showing me photos of someone else's surgery, explained that the larger nerves were encased in something like a sheath, and that there was essentially no reason to fear that they would be injured.

We also discussed the area of my previously extracted upper right wisdom tooth. Although the cavitat test had shown no problem in that area, Dr. Kulacz said that my panorex x-ray seemed to suggest that there might be a cavitation in that area as well. As he was concerned, he offered to check out that area also at no extra cost to me, and we agreed that this was the wise thing to do.

The general anesthesia was performed by an anesthesiologist whom Dr. Kulacz highly trusts and respects. The experience of the surgery during anesthesia was somewhat like a pleasant dream. After the IV was inserted, I began to feel sleepy, and before I knew it, I was barely conscious of anything except perhaps a vague sound of drilling. Then the next thing I knew, the surgery, which had really lasted about 3 hours, was over.

Dr. Kulacz seemed quite happy about the surgery even though he had found quite large cavitations; he had been able to successfully remove much of the infection in my jaw. He had found a large cavitation even in the upper right jaw, the area that had shown only a suggestion of a problem on the x-ray. We were so glad that we had decided to check out that area in addition to the more obvious ones.

Healing from the surgery took place quickly and easily. I fully expected to need painkillers after the anesthesia lost its effect, but the pain was so minimal that I didn't need any. Thirteen days after the surgery I went to my local dentist to have the sutures removed. He and his assistant both seemed surprised that I had healed so well already. I also went to a clinic in Switzerland the following month and the doctor there also exclaimed, "Good job!" when he looked in my mouth.

-C.H., Pennsylvania

Congestive Heart Failure

L.M. of Armonk, New York had a heart attack at age 40, a second heart attack nine years later that was treated with coronary bypass surgery. When he came to my office at age 62 he was in congestive heart failure and awaiting a heart transplant. He presented with severe periodontal disease as well as chronic endodontic infections. After the extraction of his root canal-treated teeth and the effective treatment of his periodontal disease, his cardiac status improved enough that he was no longer considered a transplant candidate.

Headache and Sinus Congestion

C.C. of Ridgefield, Connecticut presented with a constant headache for one year duration as well as chronic sinus congestion in the left sinus. Both his dentist and an ear, nose, and throat specialist found no pathology or cause for his condition. After removing tooth #14 which was treated with a root canal, both his headaches and sinus congestion were immediately alleviated.

Microscopic pathologic analysis of samples from the patient above found that cross sections through the apical portions of the roots displayed abundant necrotic (dead) debris adjacent to endodontic materials in two apical canals, with chronic inflammatory cells in one canal. The diagnosis: Nonsuppurative pulpal necrosis of endodontically treated tooth and a periapical granuloma with chronic nonsuppurative osteomyelitis of surrounding bone. The full pathology report on tissues obtained from the patient appears in Appendix E.

Hearing Loss and Sinus Infection

To: Dr. George Meinig, C/O Bion Publishing
P.O. BOX 10, Ojai, CA 93024
January 28, 2002

Dear Dr. Meinig:
I just wanted to take the time to thank you first of all for writing such an informative

book, Root Canal Cover-Up. It really made me even more aware of the possible connection between my poor health and my root canals. Even though the sad journey started for me over 10 years ago when I had my first root canal, I am thankful that the worst is over. I am now root canal free. I had a total of three removed all were infected.

I was suffering from severe stomach problems that started months after my first root canal. I was even hospitalized for Pancreatitis. The 7-day hospital stay cost over $25,000 and none of the specialists could find out what was causing the symptoms. They gave me medicine to relieve the symptoms but never could get to the root of the cause.

As you can see as you read my health history, it took several more years but finally I did find relief. I hope my body can fully recover from the years of infection and leeching metals. Right now I feel better than I have in years.

And that brings me to my final reason for this letter. I really want to thank you for referring me to Dr. Robert Kulacz. He was brave and skilled enough to venture into my sinus cavity and clean out the infection. He told me on the day of the surgery that if the infection returned that it was because there was a secondary infection in my upper sinus area that he could not reach. He said the ENT Doctor would eas-

ily be able to help me with any residual infection. But that was not necessary, Dr. Kulacz cleaned the area so thoroughly that he must have gotten all the infection because it has not returned. So thanks again for the referral, for your book, and for having the integrity to tell the truth.

-G.R.B., Rahway, NJ

CC: Dr. Robert Kulacz

The following health history was provided to Dr. Kulacz by G.R.B.

Discussed issue with my dentist (who performed the last 2 root canals):

1. *He admitted that the horrible stench in my mouth (I smelled it when he inserted rubber dam) was due to bacteria from my root canals.*

2. *Yet, he refused to believe that the same bacteria was causing my stomach problems. Therefore, he refused to remove root canalled teeth. Referred me to a root canal specialist.*

3. *Specialist said root canals looked good on X-ray. But could not say for certain that bacteria was not causing my problem. Requested to be informed if once root canals were removed my symptoms improved.*

One Week After Surgery:

A Miracle! The sinus infection is gone. No traces of it, and I feel wonderful. I am finally symptom free, with no root canals in my mouth,

Still partially deaf in left ear, I believe this will always serve as a reminder to me of just how dangerous to one's health root canals can be.

CHAPTER TWELVE

BEYOND *Root Canal Treatment*

Hidden Gangrene: The Cavitation

What is a Cavitation?

While the title of this chapter may seem a bit alarming and even a bit incredible, it is no exaggeration. A cavitation is a residual hole or defect in the jawbone at the site of an old, or "healed" tooth extraction. The contents of a cavitation typically consist of toxins, osteomyelitic and osteonecrotic (dead) bone, the presence of microbes, and various types of tissue fragments. Histologically, cavitation contents have distinct similarities to wet gangrene.

Cavitations are Common

It is a fact that cavitations are very commonly found in most people who have had tooth extractions; the vast majority of dental patients have one or more of them. The statistical incidence of cavitations was first presented in the winter 1996 issue of the *Journal of Advancement in Medicine*. In a review of 112 patients who were explored for possible cavitations, it was found that nearly 90% (313 out of 354) of wisdom tooth extraction sites had cavitated.[1] Many of these cavitations were not at recent extraction sites. Typically, years and often decades had passed since the teeth had been extracted. All of the other extraction sites also demonstrated the ability to cavitate, although the incidence of cavitation lessened as the size of the teeth extracted became smaller or as the amount of infection present at the time of extraction was less. The bigger the hole and more pronounced the infection, the more likely that healing would be incomplete and remain incomplete. Once present, cavitations tend to remain; they will never heal spontaneously. Complete surgical debridement is required in order to get new, healthy bone to fill in the defect. Cavitations do not heal on their own without surgical intervention, no matter how much time is allowed.

Why Cavitations Develop

An important reason that cavitations develop is due to the nature of the standard extraction technique. The typical technique does not always remove the periodontal ligament and may not allow adequate blood flow through the cortical bone of the tooth socket to initiate new bone formation.

The tooth socket is a dense layer of cortical bone designed to withstand the forces of chewing. The tooth is held in place within the socket by the periodontal ligament. The periodontal ligament is a thin yet dense connective tissue layer that lines the socket, anchors the tooth to the cortical bone, and acts as a shock absorber to cushion the forces of chewing.

Oftentimes after extraction, the periodontal ligament remains attached to the cortical bone of the tooth socket. When the tooth is extracted but the periodontal ligament remains, the surrounding bone has no physiological awareness that the tooth is gone. The body may not initiate resorption of the periodontal ligament and cortical tooth socket bone, and new bone formation may not occur. Instead, only a small amount of new bone grows at the top of the extraction site, where the ligament ends, and the typical thin cap of bone over the extraction site results. Because new bone

When the tooth is extracted but the periodontal ligament remains, the surrounding bone has no physiological awareness that the tooth is gone.

and the associated blood vessel plexus have failed to form, the bacteria introduced to the extraction site remain within the cavitation, creating a site of focal infection with the associated toxin release. Bone samples from the perimeter of the cavitation sent for microscopic analysis show both chronic osteomyelitis and osteonecrosis.

Because new bone and the associated blood vessel plexus have failed to form, the bacteria introduced to the extraction site remain within the cavitation, creating a site of focal infection.

Dentists should completely remove the periodontal ligament lining the tooth socket. If the extraction is due to periodontal disease or the tooth is a root canal-treated tooth, complete removal of the cortical bone socket is recommended in order to expose healthy, bleeding medullary bone. At the very least, the periodontal ligament should be removed, and a large number of closely spaced perforations through the cortical bone socket should be made with a burr to induce bleeding. This increased blood flow will increase the likelihood that the osteoclast cells will completely resorb the tooth socket and the osteoblast cells will initiate new bone formation. Failure of the cortical bone of the socket to resorb will produce the appearance on X-ray called laminar rain.

Historical Perspective on Cavitations

Although still not recognized by modern dentistry to be the common and toxic entity that it is, the cavitation was actually described as far back as 1915 by the dental pioneer, G. V. Black. While Dr. Black did not call what he found a "cavitation," he nevertheless described very accurately the pathology and gross appearance as is described today. Dr. Black considered bone necrosis to be typical of the cavitation lesion and to be the ongoing factor that resulted in the hollowed-out area so often found at the site of an old extraction. The gradual death of bone produces a softening of the area until it eventually results in an actual hole.

Dr. Black labeled this process "chronic osteitis," even though he did not completely understand how such extensive internal bone destruction could occur without obvious external signs of inflammation and swelling. He also noted that the patient was not typically acutely ill, and did not present with symptoms such as fever. Even though Dr. Black realized that the absence of such classical inflammation/infection-associated signs and symptoms flew in the face of standard medical and dental knowledge, he still recognized the existence of these lesions and advocated that they should be thoroughly debrided.

It is known that some disease-causing micro-organisms such as mycoplasma do not present with the classic signs and symptoms of infection normally seen on blood tests or clinical evaluation. These "silent" infections often go initially undetected by our standard laboratory tests and can later cause and/or promote the development of various chronic diseases. Even when such a disease becomes well-established, the possibility of occult, or hidden, infection is rarely entertained as a likely cause of the disease or even as a significant contributory factor in its development. Likewise, cavitations are chronically infected and toxic lesions that can also go undetected by standard tests and yet play a substantial role in the initiation and maintenance of chronic disease, especially when the bone necrosis continues to spread to previously healthy bone.

In his surgical approach to cavitation debridement, Dr. Black noted that it was usually easy to enter the thin cap of bone at the old extraction site and then proceed to remove all of the contents and softened, diseased bone until solid bone margins were reached.

Even though Dr. Black was a dental pioneer who is still held in high esteem by dentists today (he is known as the "father of operative dentistry"), his findings on cavitations never were incorporated into current dental thought or dental teaching. There is no way to know whether this omission was deliberate or inadvertent. Regardless of this oversight, the appreciation of the existence of cavitations by other dental authors once again emerged in the 1970s. Much of this writing associated cavitations with undiagnosed facial pain syndromes, and the literature began to talk about "NICO," or neuralgia-inducing cavitational osteonecrosis. Neuralgia refers to pain extending along the pathway of one or more nerves. Patients who presented with trigeminal neuralgias and other atypical facial neuralgias were often found to have cavitations at old extraction sites. After the cavitations were properly debrided, many of these patients experienced resolution of their pain.

> *Much of this writing [from recent dental authors] associated cavitations with undiagnosed facial pain syndromes.*

The scientific literature has also labeled cavitations with several other names. In addition to NICO, they have also been referred to as Ratner, Roberts, or trigger point bone cavities, as well as alveolar cavitational osteopathosis. But regardless of the name, the entity remains the same, although the clinical consequences can vary widely among the afflicted patients.

Diagnosing Cavitations

While cavitations can occur in anybody, the work-up should always include an evaluation of the multiple initiating and predisposing risk factors for the development of a cavitation. A comprehensive oral examination should then be performed. Many (but not all) cavitations of the upper jaw can be detected by discomfort elicited by direct palpation (finger pressure on the bone). Upper jaw cavitations are easier to detect than lower jaw cavitations by palpation due to the differing bone densities of the upper and lower jaws. If the cavitation is near the surface of the bone, pain may be elicited when pressure is applied to the tissue directly overlying the area.

Sometimes cavitations or even root canal-treated teeth can cause referred pain to the head and other parts of the body such as the shoulder, hip, or knee. Root canal-treated teeth can share this ability with cavitations since the tissue specimen found in the socket of a freshly extracted root canal-treated tooth can have similar characteristics to the contents of a cavitation with regard to toxins, bacteria, and evidence of osteonecrosis and chronic osteomyelitis. In fact, almost any area of the body can experience referred pain from a cavitation or a root canal-treated tooth.

Cavitations that produce facial neuralgias form the syndrome called NICO, already mentioned above. Sometimes NICO sites can also cause referred pain to distant sites in the body. Just as a heart attack can frequently cause referred pain to the jaw and left arm, cavitations can cause referred pain as well. However, it is very important to realize that most of the time there is no associated referred pain with cavitations and root canal-treated teeth. Furthermore, when referred pain at some remote site of the body is present, the site of the cavitation itself is still frequently pain-free. This referred pain will only resolve after the cavitation has been surgically debrided or the root canal-treated tooth has been extracted and the extraction site properly debrided in a similar fashion.

> *Cavitations that produce facial neuralgias form the syndrome called NICO... Sometimes NICO sites can also cause referred pain to distant sites in the body.*

A diagnostic test to determine any link between the area where pain is felt and the cavitation can be performed by injecting a non-vasoconstrictor anesthetic near the site of the cavitation.

If the referred pain goes away or is significantly diminished after injection of the local anesthetic, it is probable that the cavitation is the cause of the referred pain.

Sometimes the referred pain does not go away when local anesthetic is placed near the cavitation. This does not necessarily mean that the cavitation is still not the source of the referred pain. Factors such as decreased blood supply to the bone and lack of adequate access of the anesthesia to the area most responsible for generation of the pain may prevent relief of symptoms. Surgical intervention may still produce positive results, although pain might sometimes persist. Diagnostic confirmation should always be attempted when referred pain is suspected.

Nevertheless, all suspected cavitation sites should be explored and properly debrided if possible, regardless of the presence or absence of associated symptomatology, as it is always desirable to clean out dead and infected tissue wherever it might be present in the body. An asymptomatic cavitation can always progress and evolve to a larger, symptomatic one.

As mentioned earlier, it needs to be emphasized that only a small percentage of cavitations produces either local or referred pain. This does NOT mean that these cavitations are toxin-free and incapable of potentially affecting other parts of the body. The toxicity test devised by Boyd Haley, PhD, has found all cavitation samples tested thus far to be toxic, with most of them proving to be very highly toxic. This same test found similar toxins in the 5,000+ consecutive extracted root canal-treated teeth that he tested (see Chapter Three).

All suspected cavitation sites should be explored and properly debrided if possible... as it is always desirable to clean out dead and infected tissue wherever it might be present in the body.

How these toxins affect an individual will depend upon many factors including genetic susceptibility, immune system function, and the degree of access that the toxins have to the rest of the body. Root canal-treated teeth may disseminate their toxins throughout the body and impact health negatively, while a single small cavitation may have little to no substantive clinical impact. Conversely, multiple and/or large cavitations in a patient can contribute to a wide variety of advanced chronic degenerative diseases. The bottom line is that all cavitations should be completely debrided, unless some unique clinical circumstance or individual risk/benefit concern indicates otherwise.

X-Raying the Invisible?

The diagnostic tool that has been most used to diagnose cavitations is the panoramic dental X-ray. This large X-ray includes the upper jaw, lower jaw, teeth and sinuses. Sometimes a smaller periapical X-ray that focuses on the root of a tooth or a limited area of the jawbone is used to get a closer view of a particular area. Although many lesions can be seen on a panoramic X-ray, it does not reliably depict areas of bone in the beginning stages of osteonecrosis, or cavitation formation. Many times these lesions do not show up on X-ray until there is a 50% deterioration of the bone density relative to adjacent normal bone. This is due to the anatomical nature of bone, which is literally a substance comprised of multiple small holes superimposed upon each other and sandwiched between denser outer bone coverings. Remember that an X-ray is a two-dimensional picture of a three-dimensional object.

These lesions may take on a variety of X-ray appearances. One appearance is a dark space of variable size, indicating a relatively larger hole or space in the bone than is usually present within normal bone.

When a cavitation is surgically explored, it is common to "fall into" a hole in the bone after very little drilling through the thin cap of bone typically covering the cavitation. The bone surrounding these holes tends to be ischemic, contributing to the failure of the bone to fully heal. With marginal blood supply, the hole itself may have little, and sometimes no bone covering it, just the layer of gingiva (gum tissue) covering the hole.

Even though the X-ray remains the tool most commonly used to visualize a cavitation, it is very important to know that an X-ray is generally sub-optimal for this application. Many times a cavitation will not be seen on an X-ray, except by a highly experienced surgeon with an extensive background in working with and diagnosing cavitations.

Because they are difficult to consistently image on X-ray, cavitations have been labeled the "invisible osteomyelitis." Practically speaking, what this also means is that an X-ray in which no cavitation is clearly visualized can NEVER be used as the sole reason for concluding that a cavitation is not present. In other words, *a positive X-ray picture can rule IN the presence of a cavitation, but a negative, normal-appearing X-ray picture can never rule OUT the presence of a cavitation.* Even some dentists who are very aware of the presence of cavitations persist in concluding that they cannot be present in a patient who has a normal-appearing panoramic dental X-ray. This approach will *always* miss more cavitations than it finds. The increased utilization of 3D X-ray imaging is improving cavitation diagnosis.

Physical Appearance and Characteristics of Cavitations

The physical appearance of the contents of cavitations can vary widely. Sometimes cavitations are composed of very mushy bone that can contain scattered globules of fat, with an overall likeness to chicken soup without the fat being skimmed. Cavitation contents may also have a sawdust-like appearance. The contents can even resemble melted chocolate ice cream. Colors described include green, yellow-green, or tarry black. Sometimes the contents are even clear. Consistencies of the contents range from clumps resembling cottage cheese to a loose, runny liquid. Distinctive unpleasant odors are sometimes present. Sometimes a sulfurous, "rotten egg" smell is present. Any odor that is associated with tissue breakdown and death secondary to chronic anaerobic bacterial growth and toxicity can occur. Interestingly, the dentist will sometimes miss the smell, but the patient will not.

The degree of development of a cavitation inside the jawbone can vary significantly from one patient to the next. Depending on a number of local and systemic factors, the progressive cellular death of bone tissue as described long ago by Dr. Black can proceed largely unchecked, or it can "stall out" after only a relatively small cavitation has formed. Because of this, the actual configurations of cavitations inside the jawbone vary widely. They can be very focal and virtually impossible to delineate from the adjacent "normal" holes found in non-diseased, cancellous bone. They can also be quite large, in the range of one centimeter in length or even more. Fingerlike projections can evolve, and the overall cavitation can develop an "amoeba-like," amorphous appearance. Sometimes they are rounded and sometimes they are very ragged and irregular along their boundaries. On occasion, the boundaries will calcify to a degree, and the ability for such a cavitation to show up on X-ray will be greatly enhanced.

When a patient has had consecutive teeth extracted, or is completely edentulous (without teeth), it is very common for cavitations to extend to a degree such that interconnections among them are formed. These progress to the point that some patients who have had all of their teeth extracted will actually have a tubular defect throughout much of their jawbone containing exceptionally large amounts of the toxic cavitation contents. This is referred to as a "channel cavitation." This is also why many patients who have few or no teeth can have as much or more dental toxicity as patients with many remaining teeth. Many edentulous patients are dealing with an enormous amount of toxicity on a daily basis from their extensive cavitation disease.

Risk Factors for Cavitation Development

Bisphosphonates. Bisphosphonate drugs are used in the treatment of osteopenia and osteoporosis. These drugs inhibit the bone-resorbing osteoclast cells. Normally, bone is continually resorbed by osteoclasts and new bone formed by osteoblasts. When the balance of bone resorption to bone formation is negatively altered, more bone will be resorbed than is formed, and the bone will become less dense. The end result of this process is osteoporosis. Bisphosphonates alter osteoclast function, significantly slowing down bone resorption. Unfortunately, we need bone resorption to remove the residual tooth socket bone to allow the tooth socket to properly heal and fill in with new medullary bone. Bisphosphonates significantly increase the likelihood of cavitation formation.

Clotting disorders. People with underlying blood clotting disorders are more prone to cavitations simply because blood flow to the extraction site can be compromised (see Appendix C).

Vasoconstrictors in local anesthetics. Dentists often use local anesthetics with vasoconstrictors. Vasoconstrictors such as epinephrine constrict blood vessels. They are used to both keep the local anesthetic in the area for a longer period of time and to reduce bleeding. If blood supply to the bone is already compromised by factors such as a clotting disorder, infection, previous trauma, etc., the use of a local anesthetic containing a vasoconstrictor might induce enough ischemia to the bone to cause some cell death, resulting in osteonecrosis.

Further, direct injection of local anesthetic into the bone under pressure as is used in a periodontal ligament tooth injection or an intra-osseous injection should never be used. The high pressure induced within the bone can constrict the capillary bed causing ischemia, and a local anesthetic that contains a vasoconstrictor only compounds the problem.

Treatment of Cavitations

Currently, the most effective method of treating cavitations is complete surgical removal of the dead, diseased, and toxin-containing bone. Appendix D details the surgical protocol for cavitation debridement. A complete protocol will also include measures to help optimize the patient's ability to grow new, healthy bone, which will eventually fill in the cavitation as fully as possible.

Too many dental practitioners advocate injecting different substances into the cavitation lesion with the hope of resolving the lesion non-surgically. One substance that has been injected into cavitations and elsewhere in the body is what is known as a Sanum remedy. The Sanum remedies used by dentists are homeopathic in nature, with the hope that so-called "interference fields" and other "blockages" of normal energy flow will be removed or minimized. However, Sanum remedies also contain and employ "apathogenic" microorganisms normally found in the body. As we have discussed earlier, both cavitations and root canal-treated teeth develop their incredible toxicities because of what happens when the normal, largely apathogenic, microbial flora of the mouth becomes trapped in the oxygen-deprived environments found in these diseased areas of the jawbone. The last thing any clinician should want to do would be to inject any amount of any kind of microorganism into a cavitation, in or around a root canal-treated tooth, or into any other area with little or no oxygen and blood supply. This is like throwing gasoline onto the fire. This method of just injecting something into a cavitation and expecting healing will always prove to be ineffective at best and harmful at worst. Once a tissue is dead, it is dead.

Even if a Sanum remedy were able to improve the "energy dynamics" of the mouth and body, the body will not be able to clean out a relatively large area of osteonecrosis and osteomyelitis without a good blood supply. Placing new microorganisms into a cavitation may well result in a "reactivation" and expansion of what had been an area that had been relatively fixed in size.

Also, even when the cavitation is not actually worsened by the Sanum remedy, the patient will lose precious time and money. Ironically, Sanum remedies are quite expensive and using them to treat a sick patient with cavitations will only result in that patient remaining sicker for a longer period. This can result in that patient also losing hope that this condition can be satisfactorily treated.

The surgical protocol for treating the cavitation should utilize proven surgical principles. Every aspect of the surgical procedure should be based on sound scientific research and established principles documented to promote good healing. To this end, a great deal of time and energy was spent researching every aspect of this surgical procedure beginning with the methods for diagnosing these cavitation lesions right down to the type of sutures used for closing the surgery site. This is not to say that the protocol that is presented in this book cannot be improved upon. In fact, as new technology and new research becomes available, these treatment procedures will undoubtedly evolve and change to keep up with new findings. However, this current protocol is quite effective, and it has proven to be successful in the resolution of cavitations. For information on the pathology of cavitations, go to www.maxillofacialcenter.com. See Appendix B for cavitation images and X-rays and see Appendix C for cavitation causes.

ADA Commends Weston Price

...before attacking him

During his many years of tireless service to dentistry, Weston A. Price (1870-1948) earned the deep respect and admiration of his peers, colleagues, and patients, and he was even highly commended in a tribute by his fellow ADA members. It was only toward the end of his life that several researchers began to attack his work that established the connection between root canal-treated teeth and systemic diseases. After the death of Dr. Price, the ADA realized the significance of his research. Determined to protect the root canal procedure, they undertook an aggressive campaign to discredit his invaluable contributions.

At the beginning of *Dental Infections, Oral and Systemic*, the publisher presents a posthumous biography and reproduces the tribute given to Dr. Price by the Ohio chapter of the ADA in May of 1941. A

portion of that biography and the ADA tribute is reproduced here:

> Weston Price, DDS, MS, FACD received his predoc-
> toral training in his native Canada before entering
> the University of Michigan. He received his DDS
> there in 1893. By 1900 he had published on tech-
> niques of electrically infusing tissues with anes-
> thetic, the use of X-rays in dentistry, and a broad
> spectrum of research on the use of wax patterns
> and investments for use in making gold castings.
> His pioneering work on the physical character-
> istics of gold and its alloys during the heating
> and cooling probably stimulated his interest in
> founding the first research institute for dentistry
> in the USA.
>
> Dr. Price devoted more than half of his daily
> time as Director of the Research Institute of the
> National Dental Association for over 14 years. The
> tremendous amount of research he conducted
> during that time (involving thousands of patients
> and tens of thousands of rabbits) gained him
> a position of high popularity as a speaker and
> publisher internationally. Of the over 220 papers
> and 3 major books that he authored during his
> lifetime, most of the basis was founded at the
> research Institute. He refused any salary for this
> dedicated service.
>
> During his research at the Institute, Dr. Price
> published 25 articles on the subject of the effects
> of root filled teeth on systemic diseases. Later, in
> what he considered a condensed version, these
> findings were published in two classic publica-
> tions, the 700 page *Dental Infections, Oral and*

Systemic, and its companion, the 400 plus page *Dental Infections and the Degenerative Diseases*.

Dr. Price was received readily and with respect by medical, dental, and lay audiences, As a demonstration of respect, the American Dental Association and his home Ohio contingency honored him for his outstanding contributions to the art and science of Dentistry. A "Tribute" was presented to Price in Ohio. It read:

In recognition of...

his indomitable spirit

his glowing personality

his cheerful disposition

his indefatigable energy

his innumerable written contributions to dental literature-to-medical literature- and to lay literature

his countless oral contributions to dental audiences-to-medical audiences and to lay groups

his many instructive and entertaining health radio presentations

his mechanical contribution to our profession

his electrical contributions to the art of practice

his therapeutic contributions to operative dentistry

his dietetic enlightenment

his research on physical properties of our necessary materials

his research on Foci of infection and his tireless attention to the subject of Dental Caries Research.

In recognition of these distinguished services and of his esteemed membership and friendship, the Cleveland Dental Society hereby dedicates its Spring Clinic meeting of May 1941 to the honor of Weston A. Price.

The Tribute was signed by 27 past presidents, and the current president.

This tribute is of particular significance because it clearly demonstrates the level of professional respect that the dental community had for Dr. Price. Only when the ADA eventually realized how his meticulous research threatened the very acceptance of the root canal procedure did it transform Dr. Price from dental pioneer to pariah.

Seeing is Believing: Photos Tell the Story

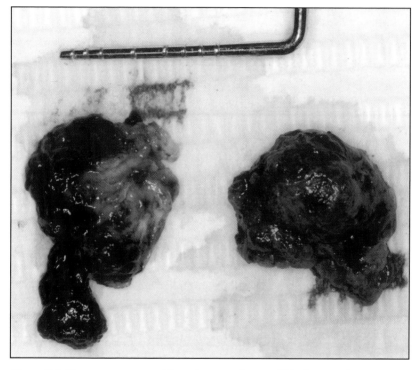

Figure B-1: Tissue mass removed from the posterior mandible (lower jaw). Panoramic X-ray of this area showed similar appearance as seen in the X-ray on page 300. Although sometimes an empty hole, cavitations can also contain fibrous and inflammatory tissue. This patient presented with facial pain for 9 years and was told by her dentist that there was "nothing wrong with her jaw." After surgical debridement this patient was pain free.

Photo: Robert Kulacz, DDS

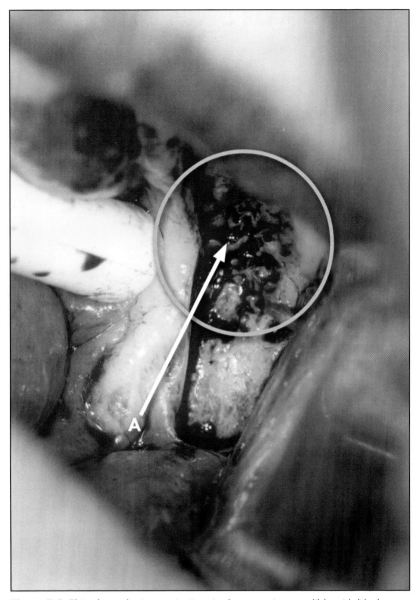

Figure B-2: This photo depicts cavitations in the posterior mandible with black, tarry tissue (A) instead of healthy, healed bone. Photo of a sagittal section cadaver mandible on page 294 illustrates how this pathology can extend throughout the jawbone.

Photo: Robert Kulacz, DDS

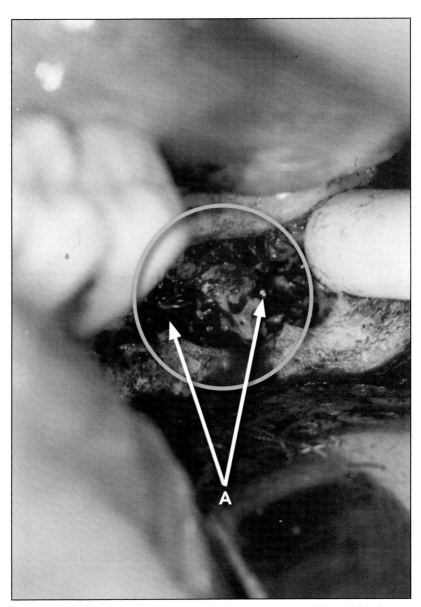

Figure B-3: This photo depicts cavitations in the posterior mandible with black, tarry tissue (A) instead of healthy, healed bone. Photo of a sagittal section cadaver mandible on page 294 illustrates how this pathology can extend throughout the jawbone.

Photo: Robert Kulacz, DDS

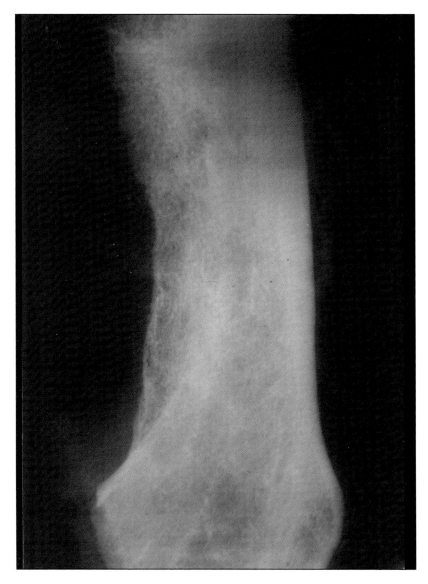

Figure B-4: This is a perfectly normal appearing X-ray of the mandible. As discussed, 2D X-rays can appear perfectly normal even though there is significant pathology in the medullary bone. This is because it takes approximately 50 percent decalcification of the medullary bone to become visible on 2D X-ray.

Photo: J.E. Bouquot, DDS, MSD

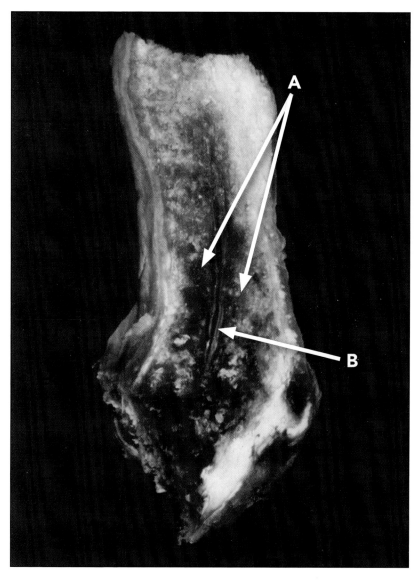

Figure B-5: This is a sagittal section of the same mandible shown in the 2D X-ray (Figure B-4). Notice the prevalence of osteonecrotic bone (A) is completely invisible on the X-ray in figure B-4 on page 292. (B) points to the neurovascular bundle.

Photo: J.E. Bouquot, DDS, MSD

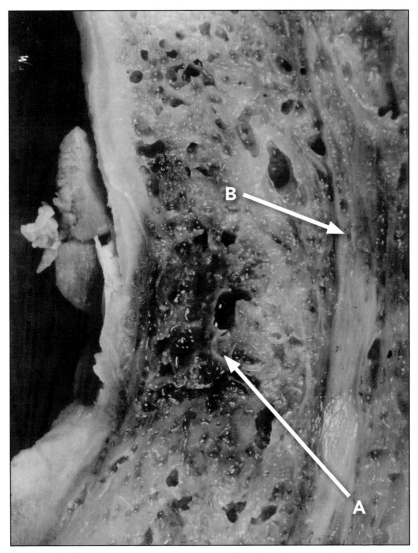

Figure B-6: This is a photo of a cadaver mandible (lower jaw) that is split in sagittal section (front to back). This person had severe facial pain due to ischemic osteonecrosis/chronic osteomyelitis that involved a large part of the lower jaw (A) including the neurovascular bundle (B). Any infection or toxin release would have an easy pathway to the rest of the body via the large blood vessels that pass through this diseased bone.

Photo: J.E. Bouquot, DDS, MSD

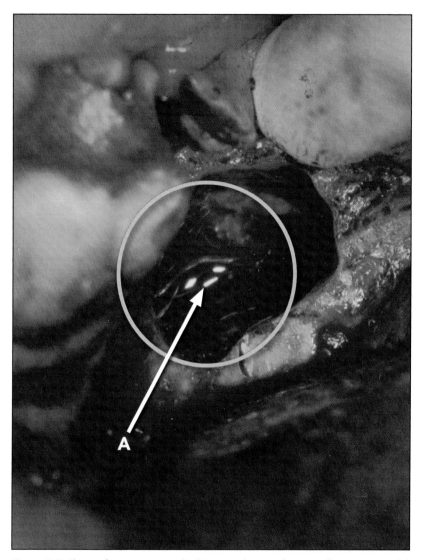

Figure B-7: Photo of a cavitation in the lower wisdom tooth area. There was no solid bone at this site, and the inferior alveolar neurovascular bundle (main nerve and blood vessels) can be seen at the base of the cavitation.

Photo: J.E. Bouquot, DDS, MSD

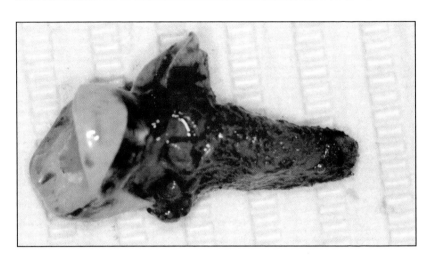

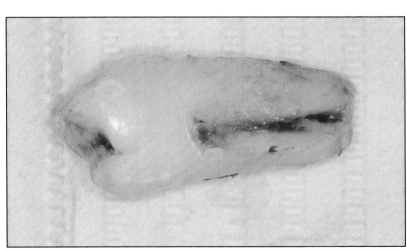

Figure B-8: Tooth on the left is a healthy premolar tooth extracted for orthodontic reasons. Note the healthy color and lack of inflammatory tissue around the root.

Figure B9: Tooth on the right is a root canal-treated tooth that is blackened at the root apex. The jawbone around the apex of this tooth was also black and mushy with a diagnosis of chronic osteomyelitis and a positive microbiology culture of two anaerobic bacteria species.

Photos: Robert Kulacz, DDS

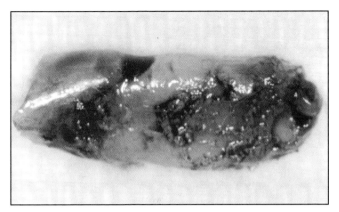

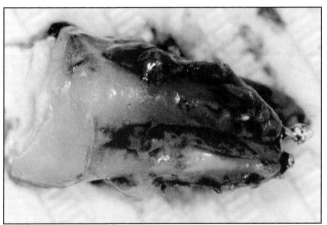

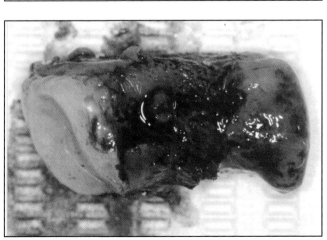

Figure B-10: These are three root canal-treated teeth. Notice the discoloration and inflammatory tissue attached to the root. These roots are in the jawbone where bacteria and exotoxins can readily migrate into the body. Compare these to the non-infected tooth in Figure B-8 on page 296 that was extracted for orthodontic purposes.

Photos: Robert Kulacz, DDS

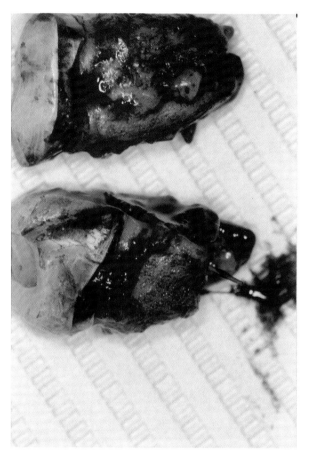

Figure B-11: Tooth on the left was the worst smelling root canal-treated tooth that I ever extracted. Note the severe dark discoloration of the entire root and the ball of infection around the end of the root.   Photo: Robert Kulacz, DDS

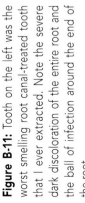

Figure B-12: Two root canal-treated teeth. Note the large amount of red inflammatory tissue around these roots and the silver point filling material protruding out from the broken root. Silver point root canal fillings cannot conform to the shape of the root canal space and are inferior to gutta-percha root canal filling. Although not routinely used, we wonder how many root canal-treated teeth have this type of root canal filling. These teeth were extremely toxic.

Photo: Robert Kulacz, DDS

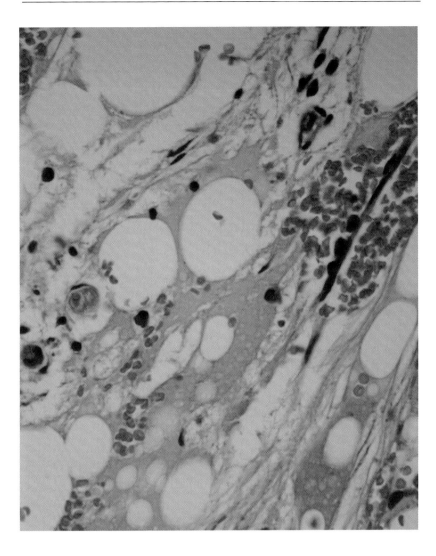

Figure B-13: Bone marrow edema in NICO lesion. The most diagnostic feature is a diffuse, pink, thick "serous ooze" (also called plasmostasis) with loose, embedded fat cells (large oval white/clear spaces in the photo); this is a protein-rich fluid pushed out of the marrow vessels by increased pressures. Clustered free or extravasated erythrocytes represent hemorrhage from focal microinfarcts. More than 72% of NICO patients have one or more inherited hypercoagulation states with increased risk of throwing small clots.

Photo: J.E. Bouquot, DDS, MSD

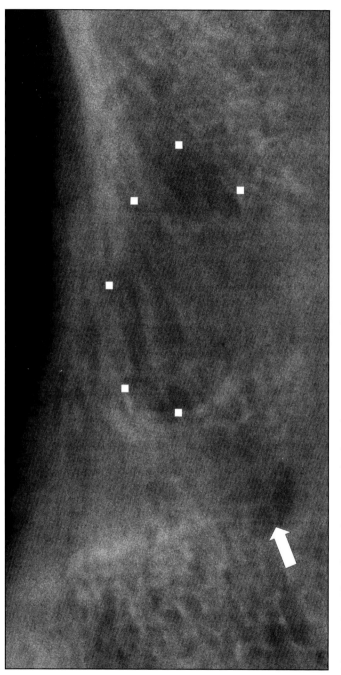

Figure B-14: White dots outline a completely void or empty region of bone, i.e. ischemic bone cavitation, in a patient with idiopathic pain of the left mandible. The arrow points to the mental foramen, above which is an inverted triangle-shaped residual socket. The crestal bone above the socket was missing, replaced by a thick fibrous scar tissue; the overlying mucosa was normal in appearance.

Photo: J.E. Bouquot, DDS, MSD

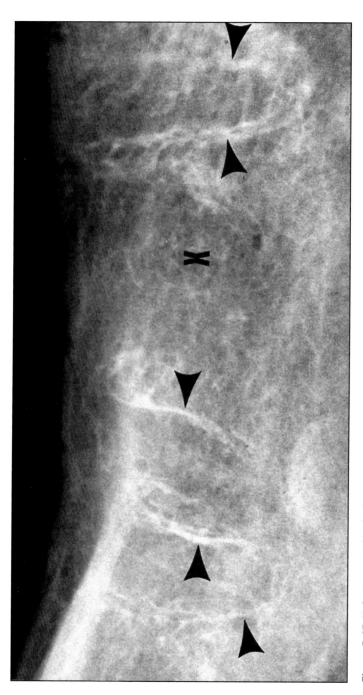

Figure B-15: X depicts a void in the bone (cavitation) and arrows point to residual tooth socket (laminar rain) that failed to resorb. Normal healing occurs with resorption of the tooth socket and deposition of new bone in the extraction space.

Photo: J.E. Bouquot, DDS, MSD

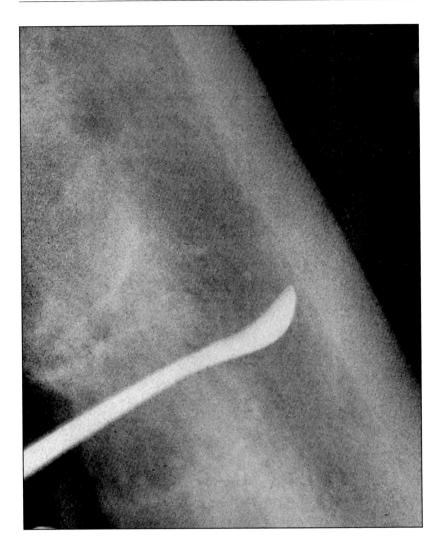

Figure B-16: Several rounded and partially remodeled residual sockets remain years after extraction in a patient with severe local pain of 3 years duration. The crestal bone was missing in the premolar area, replaced by a thin, partially perforated fibrous tissue. Beneath the fibrous tissue was a bony void, i.e. ischemic bone cavitation. A curette has been placed into the void prior to taking the radiograph.

Photo: J.E. Bouquot, DDS, MSD

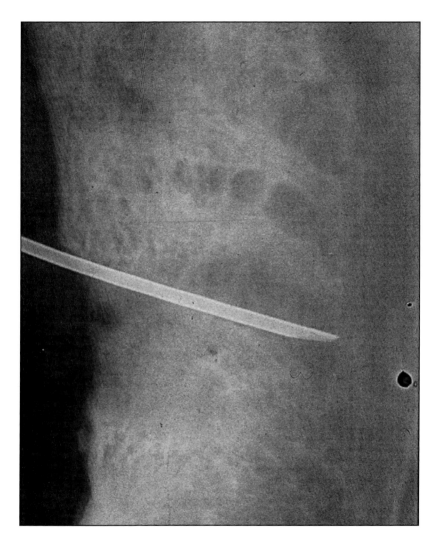

Figure B-17: Multiple residual sockets are visible in the right mandibular molar region; one shows so little remodeling that even the Jacob's ladder pattern remains between the first molar roots (on right). The second molar site was covered not with bone but with discolored fibrous tissue. The surgeon pushed a needle through the fibrous tissue and it literally fell into a void or ischemic bone cavitation beneath. The teeth had been removed decades earlier and the patient had suffered from local "idiopathic" pain for almost the entire time.

Photo: J.E. Bouquot, DDS, MSD

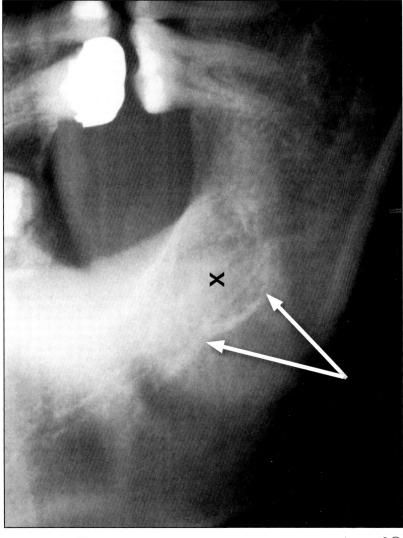

Figure B-18:

Intramedullary fibrous scar. A large, bilobed, slightly radiolucent lesion of the right mandibular third molar and ramus region has a sclerotic rim surrounding much of it. At surgery the area was found to be filled with very dense, avascular collagen, i.e. fibrous scar tissue. Such scar tissue is almost unheard of outside of the jaws and when in the jaws may be associated with considerable pain; it usually doesn't show sclerosis of the borders. Arrows point to the sclerotic borders of the cavitation (X)

Photo: J.E. Bouquot, DDS, MSD

Causes of Cavitations and Associated Conditions

Overview of Causes

Cavitation disease, or ischemic osteonecrosis, results from both systemic and local problems at a number of sites in the body. Although not so much a disease in it own right, ischemic osteonecrosis is the localized result of anything which significantly reduces the blood flow through the bone marrow.

Ischemic osteonecrosis of the head of the femur was once called "coronary disease of the hip" because of the associated marrow ischemia (reduced blood flow) and infarction (death of tissue from too little to no blood flow).

In cases of ischemic osteonecrosis involving the femoral head, the list of diseases and biological phenomena capable of producing this damage has continued to grow. Some of the etiologic factors are much more significant than others. Some factors are primary causes and other factors act as triggering mechanisms or "second hits" in persons otherwise susceptible to bone marrow blood flow problems.

Jaws are especially susceptible to cavitations and ischemic osteonecrosis for several reasons. The jaws are especially susceptible to reduced blood flow problems. Trauma and infection are the primary triggering events for osteonecrosis, and no other bones come close to the level of trauma and infection experienced by the jaws being subjected to an array of insults including: tooth and gum infections, tooth extractions, trauma (like a fist to the face), and oral or root canal (endodontic) or gum (periodontic) surgery.

Another cause of osteonecrosis can be added to those mentioned above, which is rather unique to dental procedures: the local anesthetics used to numb the jaw for tooth procedures or oral surgery. These drugs often contain powerful chemicals (vasoconstrictors, e.g. epinephrine) designed to drastically reduce the blood flow in the area, thereby keeping the anesthetic in place longer and allowing more time to work.

These anesthetics are wonderful for the procedure itself but can be disastrous for someone with any one of the undiagnosed hypercoagulation disorders to be discussed. Moreover, the poor outflow characteristic of osteonecrosis means that the vasoconstrictor can remain in the area far longer than the few minutes needed for profound local anesthesia. And to add injury to insult, literally, the reperfusion of the bone after the vasoconstriction wears off releases large numbers of tissue-damaging reactive oxygen species. Normal tissues can withstand this onslaught nicely, but a nutrient-starved ischemic marrow does not maintain its marginal health status as well.

SPECIFIC CAUSES OF ISCHEMIC OSTEONECROSIS

Hypercoagulation States

Hypercoagulation (a state where the blood clots more readily) is common. Some of the most common initiating factors are:

✓ **Undiagnosed coagulation disorders**

The most important underlying, and almost always unappreciated, risk factor for cavitations comes from genetic coagulation disorders. Patients should be asked about a family history of clotting problems. This hypercoagulation problem might be suggested by a family history of stroke and heart attacks at an early age (less than 55 years), hip replacement or "arthritis" (especially at an early age), and deep vein thrombosis.

Hypercoagulation may be a life-threatening problem. Always keep in mind that the presence of a hypercoagulation state makes the patient susceptible to stroke, myocardial infarction, deep vein thrombosis, and other serious or life-threatening conditions. Usually a secondary problem or "triggering event" must occur, such as local infection, trauma, medications, etc.

✓ **Other associated diseases**

There are other diseases associated with hypercoagulation. These include:

- Behçet's disease
- Chronic fatigue syndrome
- Fibromyalgia
- Irritable bowel syndrome
- Sickle cell crisis
- Migraine headaches

The significance of these associations is not completely clear—direct studies are needed to prove these links—but these disorders appear to occur frequently in patients with ischemic osteonecrosis.

Hormones

✓ **Estrogen**

Estrogen replacement therapy can be a cause of osteonecrosis. Estrogen enhances coagulation. In persons with a hypercoagulation state (at least 6% of the population) the risk of thrombosis from estrogen use increases, sometimes dramatically. For example, the risk for a person with a hypercoagulation disorder of forming a clot somewhere in the body (not just the jaws) is increased by more than 80 times when estrogen replacement is given. The orthopedic literature sometimes refers to this as estrogen-related ischemic osteonecrosis.

Pregnancy is associated with increased estrogen levels. Because of this, pregnant women are at an elevated risk of developing ischemic osteonecrosis, especially of the hip. A mild, self-limiting condition that is a precursor to osteonecrosis, transient ischemic osteoporosis, often spontaneously regresses with immobility after the birth of the child. Multiple joints may be involved, sometimes moving from one to another over time (migratory ischemic osteoporosis).

✓ Hypercortisolism

Hypercortisolism (excess corticosteroid presence) is another cause of osteonecrosis. It can result from either excess natural production or from the common practice of prescribing prednisone or prednisolone to prevent swelling after oral surgical procedures. Corticosteroid use is the most common cause of non-traumatic osteonecrosis. Although the risk appears to be magnified by higher doses and longer periods of administration, there are reports of striking hip osteonecrosis from a single week's use of Medrol. The orthopedic literature contains articles pertaining to corticosteroid-induced osteonecrosis. The mechanism for this is not well-defined.

✓ **Hypothyroidism**

Low levels of thyroid hormone have been associated with increased risk of developing ischemic osteonecrosis of the hip, probably because the diminished metabolism produced by this condition reduces blood flow rates throughout the body.

Miscellaneous Factors

✓ **Autoimmunity and Hypersensitivity**
- Systemic lupus erythematosus
- Antiphospholipid syndrome

✓ **Maxillary sinus infections**

Recurring maxillary sinus infections with the potential seeding of bacteria in the alveolar bone, producing osteomyelitis (bone infection), is a major risk factor. The inflammatory mediators at work in this chronic process are capable of increasing local and systemic coagulation. This is generally not a problem for a normal person but can be, again, disastrous for the 6% of the population who have undiagnosed or "silent" hypercoagulation states.

✓ Gaucher's disease

This lipid storage disease is associated with hyperviscosity, thrombocytopenia, and decreased factor IX and protein C. It has been suggested that when the very large lesional cells, Gaucher cells, enter the blood vessels they act as emboli and when they fragment their breakdown products they trigger excess intravascular coagulation, leading to thrombosis and hemorrhage (microinfarctions). Just before a crisis, there is radioisotopic evidence of ischemia, but it may be days or several months after the acute pain onset before a biopsy will show obvious osteonecrosis.

Diseases and Conditions Associated with Osteonecrosis (any bone)

Disease or Etiologic Factor	Subcategories
Alcohol Abuse	Cirrhosis Pancreatitis
Arthritis	Subchondral cyst Subchondral marrow edema
Atmospheric Pressure Variations	Caisson's disease Deep sea diving
Blood dyscrasias	Disseminated intravascular coagulation (DIC) Sickle cell anemia

Disease or Etiologic Factor	Subcategories
Cancer	Leukemia
	Cancer-induced hypercoagulation
	Lymphoma
	Metastatic intraosseous carcinoma
	Radiation therapy for cancer
Chronic Inactivity	Bedridden
	Full body cast
	Paraplegic
Corticosteroids	Hypercortisolism
	Inflammatory bowel disease
	Lupus erythematosus
	Transplants
Estrogen	Birth control pills
	Estrogen replacement therapy
	Fertility drugs
	Pregnancy
	Prostate chemotherapy
	Transient ischemic osteoporosis
Hypercoagulable state, local	Acute infections/inflammation
	Chronic infection/ inflammation
	Increased intramedullary pressures

Disease or Etiologic Factor	Subcategories
Hypercoagulable state, systemic	Antiphospholipid antibody syndrome
	Factor V Leiden gene mutation
	Hyperhomocysteinemia
	Homozygosity for MTHFR* or CBS**
	Protein C deficiency
	Protein S deficiency
Hyperlipidemia & embolic fat	Diabetes mellitus
	Dysbaric phenomena
	Fracture of bone
	Hemoglobinopathies
	Osteomyelitis, acute
Hypersensitivity reactions	Allograft organ rejection
	Anaphylactic shock
	Immune globulin therapy
	Shwartzman reaction to endotoxin
	Transfusion reactions
Hypertension	
Hypothyroidism	
Incomplete removal of the periodontal ligament at the time of tooth extraction	

*MTHFR: methylene tetrahydrofolate reductase
**CBS: cystathionine beta-synthetase

Disease or Etiologic Factor	Subcategories
Inflammation, intraosseous	Infection, bacterial and viral
	Trauma (mild or severe)
	Autoimmunity/ hypersensitivity
Neurological damage	Brain injury/surgery
Osteoporosis	Regional or generalized
Starvation	Anorexia nervosa
Storage diseases	Gaucher's disease
Tobacco use	Tobacco smoking
Vascular occlusive disease	Atherosclerosis
Vasculitis Vasoconstriction	Local anesthesia (with vasoconstrictor)
	Raynaud's phenomenon
	Tobacco use

The above information has been reproduced, with some modifications, with permission of:

J. E. Bouquot, DDS
Director of Research, Maxillofacial Center for Education & Research
212 Tibbs Road
Morgantown, WV 26508

Adjunct Professor (Retired), Department of Diagnostic & Biomedical Sciences University of Texas School of Dentistry at Houston
Adjunct Professor, Department of Rural and Community Dentistry, School of Dentistry, West Virginia University

www.maxillofacialcenter.com

Surgical Protocol for Extractions of Root Canal-Treated Teeth and Cavitation Surgery

General Observations

Tooth extractions, especially of infected teeth such as those having received root canal treatments, and cavitation debridement are surgical procedures performed in the oral cavity that involve both the soft tissues of the mouth, such as the gingiva, and the bones of the maxilla and mandible. Strict adherence to surgical protocols, such as those practiced by orthopedic surgeons, should also apply to oral surgery procedures.

It must be remembered that dentists, as surgeons of the oral cavity, are still operating on bone. Although the mouth is a more forgiving place to operate in terms of the healing of soft tissue, infected bone is difficult to completely heal no matter where in the body it is located. With the inability to iso-late and create a sterile field when operating in the mouth, the potential to develop a post-surgical in-fection in the jawbone is always a possibility.

Furthermore, the ability of the mouth to rapidly heal soft tissue infections tends to make many den-tists feel that infected bone in the mouth will heal just as readily, which is not necessarily the case. We now know how easily cavitations develop, and the seemingly complete X-ray appearance of healing after many routine dental extractions remains an illusion. Accepted surgical procedures must be fol-lowed everywhere in the body in order to optimize the chances of complete healing and complete clini-cal recovery.

If some of the periodontal ligament remains in the tooth socket after an extraction, or there is a failure to remove all of the infection in the jawbone, the remaining hole in the jawbone may not com-pletely fill in with new bone. This void in the jaw-bone is called a cavitation and by its very nature, it can be a prolific breeding ground for the same bacteria that infected the tooth in the first place. Because they are often surrounded by intact jaw-bone, cavitations often escape X-ray detection.

Therefore, to optimize the chances of complete healing and complete clinical recovery accepted sur-gical procedures must be followed everywhere in the body—and especially in the mouth.

Oral Surgery Protocol

1) A complete patient medical and dental history, including consultation with all treating physicians, is essential before treatment is rendered. As the mouth is not isolated from the rest of the body, such a complete history is important. Nearly all dental procedures, especially surgery, have systemic, body-wide effects.

2) A thorough dental evaluation of the hard and soft tissues of the oral cavity is essential. The examination should include all necessary X-rays, along with a complete clinical exam that includes pulp vitality tests of the teeth to determine which teeth are healthy and alive and which teeth might be unexpectedly nerve-dead and non-vital. Any additional tests that may aid in diagnosis and treatment planning should also be performed. It is important to point out that pulp vitality tests are an integral part in assessing the health of the teeth that did not receive root canal treatments. A dead, non-vital tooth in the mouth can be just as serious as a root canal-treated tooth.

3) After the initial assessment of the patient's condition, a treatment plan must be established. If the treatment plan includes

extractions and/or cavitation surgery, it is important to seek a surgeon who is not only surgically skilled, but who also has the ability to deliver intravenous medicines. Intravenous sedation is often necessary, and there must also be an access for the administration of appropriate antibiotics.

4) Alternative treatments such as the injection of various remedies into the site of infection, like the bone around a root canal-treated tooth or around other infected teeth, should not be done. Similarly, no injections should be made into cavitation sites. Many of these treatments actually make the disease process worse. Furthermore, there are some dentists advocating the use of these medicaments *instead* of surgery. It is impossible to restore dead bone to live bone again with any medication. Surgery must be performed to remove all of the dead and infected bone as well as establishing adequate perfusion of blood from adjacent healthy bone into the surgical site. This is the only way healing can occur.

5) Optimally, teeth should be cleaned up about two weeks prior to surgery to reduce the amount of bacteria present in the mouth and lessen the chances of post-operative infection. Laser curettage in the sulcus around

each tooth can dramatically reduce the presence of bacteria even further.

6) General medical clearance, when appropriate, should be obtained.

7) A written informed consent signed by the patient should be obtained prior to the planned procedure. All potential complications of the procedure should be thoroughly discussed. It is preferable that a family member also participates in this consent, especially to help verify that all that has been discussed is fully understood. Consideration might be given to a videotaping of the discussion of the consent, which gives the dentist further evidence that all information was discussed and was completely understood by the patient prior to signing the consent form. With the advent of the smartphone, this can be more easily performed than ever before, and the recordings can be readily stored in computer files for easy access in the future.

8) Preoperative medications such as antibiotics should be administered.

9) The oral cavity should be cleansed with an appropriate antimicrobial agent.

10) Local anesthetic **without** a vasoconstrictor should be used. Vasoconstrictors lessen the blood flow in the injected area. Good

blood flow to the surgical site is necessary to help assure the best chances of complete healing. Even the transient vasoconstriction produced by anesthetics with a vasoconstrictor can cause enough ischemia to injure the bone and cause local cell death.

11) Surgery should be performed so that the total lesion can be removed. The surgeon must be skilled in operating around the inferior alveolar nerve (the main nerve that runs through the lower jaw) as well as operating through the sinus floor and into the sinus. Many times the lesions seen around cavitations and root canal-treated teeth are more extensive than they appear on X-ray. It is important to remove **all** of the diseased tissue. This means that the surgeon should be skilled in operating around all these anatomical structures. Otherwise, the patient should be referred to another surgeon.

12) Usually, the extraction of an infected or root canal-treated tooth requires adequate exposure of the bone surrounding the tooth for good visualization in order to access the infected areas. This is obtained by laying a "flap," which simply means that the gum tissue is gently lifted off the bone. The word "gently" is emphasized here since there is a

thin layer of tissue that lays directly adjacent to the bone called the periosteum that must be treated with care. The periosteum is the tissue that supplies the outside of the bone with nutrients, and it is also where many of the sensory fibers that can cause post-operative pain are located. It must be treated with respect and handled gently. The kinder you treat the tissue during any operation the less postoperative complications will occur, and the better healing will proceed.

13) Surgical sites should be irrigated with saline solution or antibiotic solutions that are acceptable for use in orthopedic surgery. We again must remember that we are operating on bone. Plain water should never be used and medications that have not been evaluated for use in bone elsewhere in the body should also never be used for surgical sites in the jawbone.

14) Extractions should be performed as atraumatically as possible. That means that teeth with more than one root such as molars should usually be sectioned and each root removed individually. This technique avoids fractures of the bone and is kinder to the tissues. Dentists were taught in dental school to "expand the socket" by rocking teeth back and force. The term should be "crack

the socket" because cortical bone does not stretch and any expansion is obtained by breaking the bone. This should be avoided. Surgical removal of bone when indicated is a much better option and should only be performed with a surgical handpiece (NEVER a dental drill), accompanied by copious sterile saline irrigation (not plain water). Dental drills can introduce air into the surgical site that can form an air embolism. An air embolism is a dangerous situation that can cause death. In addition, dental drills use plain water as an irrigant. This water is not sterile and is not physiologic in terms of salinity. Plain water can cause bone cells to die.

The remainer of the protocol addresses both the proper cleaning of the extracted root canal site as well as the cleaning of a cavitation.

15) The approach to cavitation surgery is basically the same as the process followed to clean out the socket where a root canal-treated tooth was extracted. After tooth extraction, access to the diseased granulation tissue and bone at the bottom of the tooth socket can be readily obtained. Access to a cavitation site is gained by making a

mid-crestal incision and reflection of a full thickness mucoperiosteal flap to the buccal side of the jawbone and extending to the mucogingival fold. Using a round burr in a surgical handpiece and with copious saline irrigation, an opening is made in the crestal bone large enough to allow complete access to the cavitation.

16) Removal of the infected and ischemic bone can be performed initially with a surgical drill at low revolutions per minute with copious irrigation. It is important to keep the temperature of the bone as cool as possible. Aggressive use of a surgical drill will cause an increase in bone temperature due to friction. The bone cells in contact with the drill will die. Dead bone cells are exactly what we are trying to remove and therefore the formation of more dead bone cells must be carefully avoided. Most of the surgical debridement should be performed by hand with surgical curettes.

17) The surgical site must be continuously flushed with an irrigation solution such as 0.9% saline solution.

18) Sometimes bone grafting or sinus closure must be performed. Be sure to discuss this with your surgeon.

19) Closure of the surgical site should be accomplished with sutures.

20) Antibiotics should be given postoperatively to prevent re-infection or systemic dissemination of existing infection.

21) Sutures should be removed in seven to ten days.

22) Patients should be instructed to keep pressure on the surgical site by gently biting on surgical gauze. This helps control bleeding as well as keeps the flap close to the bone during the initial healing phase.

23) Ice should be applied to the side of the face for twenty minutes, then removed for twenty minutes. This should be repeated throughout the entire day of surgery but should not be used the following days.

24) The day after surgery the patient should gently rinse with a mild, warm salt water solution (1/4 teaspoon of salt in an 8 oz. glass of water). This should be done three to four times per day.

Cultures for aerobic and anaerobic bacteria as well as for fungus should be obtained immediately after extraction or entry into a cavitation site to get a "clean catch" sample. A clean catch sample is a sample that consists of only tissue within the surgical site without contamination. By ensuring good isolation and surgical suction, the surgical site will be free from external contamination and the sample will only contain pathogens present within the surgical site, and will not contain pathogens that may be introduced from the rest of the mouth.

These microbiological samples must be placed in the appropriate culture tubes and the laboratory instructed to let them incubate for at least two weeks. Some of the anaerobic bacteria and fungus take a long time to grow and discarding the sample after just a few days may miss the presence of important pathogens.

Bone tissue samples should be taken from all areas of the surgical site and sent for microscopic analysis by an oral pathologist. Acute and chronic osteomyelitis, osteonecrosis, and other disorders can be determined by microscopic evaluation. The results of the microbiological cultures and tissue pathology will assist in determining the need for any further treatment such as appropriate oral or IV antibiotics.

Typical Pathology Reports

Overview

A biopsy is a tissue sample removed from the patient that is examined by a pathologist to diagnose disease. The pathologist will process the tissue samples into very thin slices that can be examined under a microscope. Sometimes these slices are stained with various dyes to allow the pathologist to more easily differentiate the different cell types in the sample.

A biopsy is important because it is difficult to impossible to determine healthy or diseased tissue just by looking at it. Microscopic examination of the tissue sample allows the pathologist to see all the different cell types present and to accurately diagnose pathology.

In our case we are mainly looking for incomplete filling of the root canal space and necrotic debris left within the canal, osteonecrosis (dead bone), osteomyelitis (infected or inflamed bone), fibrous tissue, inflammatory cells, and cancer.

Results of the biopsy not only confirm our initial diagnosis but also assist us in deciding the need for any further treatment.

A Division of The Maxillofacial Center
for Diagnostics & Research
165 Scott Avenue, Suite 101, Morgantown, WV 26508
Phone: 304-292-4429 Fax: 304-291-5649

BIOPSY REPORT #HN99-2588
Surgery date: 8/18/99
Date received: 8/23/99
Date completed: 8/31/99

SURGEON: PATIENT:
Dr. Robert Kulacz   T.D.
280 Mamaroneck Ave, STE 307   AGE (yrs.)/
       GENDER:33FD
White Plains, NY 10605
914-288-0993
Fax: 914-288-0978

SOURCE OF SPECIMEN (location): **UL #15**.
CLINICAL DIAGNOSIS/DESCRIPTION: **Pulpitis.**

GROSS DESCRIPTION OF TISSUE RECEIVED:
PART A: The specimen consists of multiple cancellous, hemorrhagic, hard and partially softened bone fragments measuring 0.7x0.4x0.2 cm in aggregation. The entire specimen is decalcified.
PART B: The specimen consists of a tooth. Sections will be submitted after decalcification.

MICROSCOPIC DESCRIPTION OF TISSUE:
PART A: Sections show globules of a gray/translucent foreign material coated by PMNs and coccal bacterial colonies. PMNs are also seen with lymphocytes in small fragments of necrotic fibrovascular tissue. There is no evidence of malignancy.
PART B: Cross sections through the apical portions of the roots show one with generalized fibrosis and moderate dystrophic calcification, with peripheral edema and considerably dilated apical veins and lymphatics. The other pulps show less fibrosis and more edema and the dilated veins are not as severely enlarged. Attached periodontal ligament fragments are unremarkable. There is no evidence of malignancy.
MICROSCOPIC DIAGNOSIS:
PART A: Consistent with subacute osteomyelitis with foreign material and bacterial colonies, maxillary left first molar area.
PART B: Chronic fibrosing and calcific pulpitis with congestion and peripheral edema (combined acute and chronic pulpitis,) maxillary left second molar.
NOTE: Although we traditionally consider pulpal edema and congestion to be evidence of acute pulpitis, it could also be evidence of a chronic outflow problem. The PART A diagnosis is presumably from area #14, but would also be consistent with a periodontal abscess if#15 had a pocket associated with it. The foreign material in PART A is consistent with endodontic materials.

PATHOLOGIST: J.E. Bouquot, D.D.S, M.S.D., Director

Surgical site was the upper left jaw where the root canal-treated first molar tooth had previously been extracted and the second molar (tooth #15) was painful. The calcification, fibrosis, and vessel edema within the root canal space are indicative of inflammation in the pulp space. The bone in the previous extraction site of tooth #14 demonstrates bacterial colonies, necrotic tissue, remnants of root canal filling material, and white blood cells, consistent with a diagnosis of sub-acute osteomyelitis. Since this bone sample came from an old extraction site, the infection initiated from the root canal-treated tooth remained in the bone long after the tooth was extracted, never resolving.

Head & Neck Diagnostic of America
A Division of The Maxillofacial Center for Diagnostics & Research
165 Scott Avenue, Suite 101, Morgantown, WV 26508
Phone: 304-292-4429 Fax: 304-291-5649

BIOPSY REPORT #HN99-3872
Surgery date: 11/18/99
Date received: 11/24/99
Date completed: 12/1/99

SURGEON: PATIENT:
Dr. Robert Kulacz   T.S.
280 Mamaroneck Avenue,   Great Meadows, NJ
Suite 307 White Plains, NY   Age/ Gender: 44F
10605   Date of Birth: 1/29/55
914-288-0993 fax 914-288-0978

SOURCE OF SPECIMEN (location): Lower left
CLINICAL DIAGNOSIS/DESCRIPTION: NICO

GROSS DESCRIPTION OF TISSUE RECEIVED:
The specimen consists of multiple irregular and partially hemorrhagic calcified tissue fragments measuring 0.4x0.4x0.3 cm in aggregation. These are decalcified as PART A. Also included is mandibular molar and bicuspid with endodontic therapy and removed crowns. These are decalcified as PART B.

MICROSCOPIC DESCRIPTION OF TISSUE:
PART A: Sections show cortical bone with mild osteoblastic activity and occasional microcracking, with only occasional missing osteocytes. There are excess cement lines, as there are in underlying thicker than normal but sparsely spaced bony trabeculae. Trabeculae also show occasional missing osteocytes. Available fatty marrow shows a generalized wispy reticular fatty degeneration with small numbers of chronic inflammatory cells and scattered mast cells. Marrow veins are dilated and one area shows a pale staining granular fat necrosis with sprinkled erythrocytes, consistent with microinfarction. There is no evidence of malignancy.

PART B: Cross sections through the apical portions of the roots show two apical canals with abundant necrotic pulpal debris adjacent to endodontic materials with one also showing moderately severe internal resorption. Attached periodontal ligament is unremarkable. There is no evidence of malignancy.

MICROSCOPIC DIAGNOSIS:
PART A: Bone marrow edema with scattered chronic inflammatory cells (variant of ischemic osteonecrosis), left mandibular second molar and first bicuspid areas.

PART B: Necrotic pulpal remnants in apical canals of endodontically treated tooth, mandibular left second molar and first bicuspid.

NOTE: Most of the necrotic debris and internal root resorption is in the molar.

PATHOLOGIST: J.E. Bouquot, D.D.S., M.S.D., Director

This patient had severe facial pain. Both root canal-treated teeth had abundant dead tissue that was left in the root canal space and never cleaned out. These teeth might have looked like "successes" on X-ray, but microscopically they failed miserably. This is why X-rays cannot determine root canal success, even to ADA standards. The associated bone had inflammatory cells present, and there was evidence of poor blood flow consistent with micro-infarcts (loss of blood supply) in the blood vessels. This pathology scenario can cause NICO.

Head & Neck Diagnostic of America
A Division of The Maxillofacial Center for Diagnostics & Research
165 Scott Avenue, Suite 101, Morgantown, WV 26508
Phone: 304-292-4429 Fax: 304-291-5649

BIOPSY REPORT #HN99-3934
Surgery date: 11/18/99
Date received: 12/1/99
Date completed: 12/7/99

SURGEON: PATIENT:
Dr. Robert Kulacz   T.S.
280 Mamaroneck Avenue,   Great Meadows, NJ
Suite 307 White Plains, NY   Age/ Gender: 44F
10605   Date of Birth: 1/29/55
914-288-0993 fax 914-288-0978

SOURCE OF SPECIMEN(location): #30
CLINICAL DIAGNOSIS/ DESCRIPTION: 1) Periapical granuloma 2) Osteonecrosis

GROSS DESCRIPTION OF TISSUE RECEIVED:
The specimen consists of three of very small and nonhemorrhagic calcified tissue fragments measuring 0.3x0.2x0.1 cm in aggregation. This portion is decalcified as PART A. Also included are two fractured molar roots which have been endodontically treated and have a yellow color and these are decalcified as PART B.

MICROSCOPIC DESCRIPTION OF TISSUE:
PART A: Sections show viable cortical bone with prominent osteoid rimming and occasional osteoblastic activity. The bone appears viable but underlying bony trabeculae are thicker than normal and show excess cement lines with scattered missing osteocytes. A fragment of moderately dense collagenic connective tissue shows a degenerated stratified squamous lining epithelium along edges and contains moderate numbers of chronic inflammatory cells. Available marrow spaces are filled with a very loose fibrosis connective tissue with dilated veins and capillaries. There is no evidence of malignancy.

PART B: Cross sections through the apical portions of the roots show abundant necrotic pulpal debris and hemorrhage in all apical canals, admixed with endodontic materials and sometimes with chronic inflammatory cells. One apical canal has only a small amount of endodontic material within it. There is no evidence of malignancy.

MICROSCOPIC DIAGNOSIS:
PART A: Chronically inflamed periapical cyst with chronic sclerosing osteomyelitis (condensing ostetitis) of surrounding bone, mandibular right first molar area.

PART B: Nonsuppurative pulpal necrosis of endodontically treated tooth, mandibular right first molar.
NOTE: The osteosclerosis here may not have been prominent enough to be obvious radiographically.

PATHOLOGIST: J.E. Bouquot, D.D.S., M.S.D., Director

Root canal-treated tooth with abundant dead tissue and inflammatory cells remaining in the canal. There is a cyst at the apex of the root and chronic sclerosing osteomyelitis of the surrounding bone. Chronic sclerosing osteomyelitis is also called condensing osteitis and is often seen associated with root canal-treated teeth. This condition is considered a variant of normal by the ADA but in fact is often a reactive bone response to chronic infection/inflammation.

Head & Neck Diagnostic of America
A Division of The Maxillofacial Center for Diagnostics & Research
165 Scott Avenue, Suite 101, Morgantown, WV 26508
Phone: 304-292-4429 Fax: 304-291-5649

BIOPSY REPORT #HN2000-1279
Surgery date: 4/4/00
Date received: 4/7/00
Date completed: 4/17/00

SURGEON: PATIENT:
Dr. Robert Kulacz   C.C.
280 Mamaroneck Avenue,   Ridgefield. CT
Suite 307 White Plains,   NY Age/ Gender: 60M
10605   Date of Birth: 3/20/40
914-288-0993 fax 914-288-0978

SOURCE OF SPECIMEN(location): #14
CLINICAL DIAGNOSIS/ DESCRIPTION: Osteonecrosis/osteomyelitis.

GROSS DESCRIPTION OF TISSUE RECEIVED: The specimen consists of multiple irregular and dirty tan calcified tissue fragments measuring 0.7x0.4x0.2 cm in aggregation. These are decalcified as PART A. Also included are three endodontically treated root tips, two with periapical soft tissue attached, and these are decalcified as PART B.

MICROSCOPIC DESCRIPTION OF TISSUE:
PART A: Sections show thick cortical and trabecular bone with occasional osteoblastic activity and with only occasional missing osteocytes. Marrow spaces show areas of reticular fatty degeneration with dilated capillaries, and some areas show a moderately dense and focally edematous fibrosis with scattered chronic inflammatory cells in moderate numbers. There is no evidence of malignancy.

PART B: Cross sections through the apical portions of the roots show abundant necrotic debris adjacent to endodontic materials in two apical canals, with chronic inflammatory cells in one canal. There is no evidence of malignancy.

MICROSCOPIC DIAGNOSIS:
PART A: Periapical granuloma with chronic nonsuppurative osteomyelitis of surrounding bone, maxillary left first molar area.

PART B: Nonsuppurative pulpal necrosis of endodontically treated tooth, maxillary left first molar.

PATHOLOGIST: J.E. Bouquot, D.D.S., M.S.D., Director

Root canal-treated tooth with abundant dead tissue still left in the root canal space after canal cleaning and filling. The granulomas around the tips of the roots caused by the initial infection still persist long after root canal completion, with associated nonsuppurative osteomyelitis of the surrounding bone.

Head & Neck Diagnostic of America
A Division of The Maxillofacial Center for Diagnostics & Research
165 Scott Avenue, Suite 101, Morgantown, WV 26508
Phone: 304-292-4429 Fax: 304-291-5649

BIOPSY REPORT #HN2001-4892
Surgery date: 4/4/00
Date received: 4/7/00
Date completed: 4/17/00

SURGEON: PATIENT:
Dr. Robert Kulacz   R.S.
280 Mamaroneck Avenue,   Mahopac, NY
Suite 307 White Plains,   NY Age/ Gender: 63M
10605   Date of Birth: 7/7/38
914-288-0993 fax 914-288-0978

SOURCE OF SPECIMEN(location): #15
CLINICAL DIAGNOSIS/ DESCRIPTION: Osteomyelitis.

GROSS DESCRIPTION OF TISSUE RECEIVED:
The specimen consists of multiple irregular and dirty tan and focal hemorrhagic soft and hard tissue fragments measuring 0.6x0.5x0.4 cm in aggregation. These are decalcified as Part A. Also included is a maxillary molar with removed crown and dilacerated roots and this is decalcified as Part B.

MICROSCOPIC DESCRIPTION OF TISSUE:
PART A: Sections show a fragment of degenerated fibrous connective tissue with infiltration by a large number of chronic inflammatory cells. One edge has a degenerated stratified squamous lining epithelium along it, with PMNs seen within and beneath this epithelium. Fragments of bone from the apparent lesional periphery show occasional missing osteocytes and show marrow spaces filled with loose fibrous tissue with myxoid degeneration and occasional scattered lymphocytes. A separate mixed bacterial colony is presumed to be surface artifact, and there is no evidence of malignancy.

PART B: Cross sections through the tooth show complete replacement of apical canal contents by endodontic materials in two apical canals, with necrotic pulpal remnants admixed with endodontic materials in one apical canal. Inflammatory cells are not seen in the canal but are numerous within the attached granulation tissue. There is no evidence of malignancy

MICROSCOPIC DIAGNOSIS:
PART A: Subacutely inflamed periapical cyst, with mild chronic nonsuppurative osteomyelitis of surrounding bone, maxillary left second molar area.

PART B: Necrotic pulpal remnants in apical canal of endodontically treated tooth, maxillary left second molar.

PATHOLOGIST: J.E. Bouquot, D.D.S., M.S.D., Director

One of the three roots in this root canal-treated tooth still contains dead tissue after root canal completion. There is a cyst around the end of this root with nonsuppurative osteomyelitis of the surrounding bone.

Conclusion

The preceding pathology reports accurately represent those from tissue samples from root canal-treated tooth extraction sites. All of these patients had been regularly seen by their dentist and no pathology was diagnosed. Yet, microscopic examination of the extracted teeth and tissue samples of the surrounding bone found definitive pathology.

Many of the root canal-treated teeth still contained dead and infected tissue. The jawbone around root canal-treated teeth as well as extraction sites where root canal-treated teeth were previously extracted showed pathology such as osteonecrosis, osteomyelitis, cysts, granulomas, bacterial colonies, and disease-fighting immune cells. These focal areas of pathology are not normal.

The patients who had facial pain and were referred to neurologists left with no explanation of cause and a diagnosis of atypical facial pain of unknown origin. However, it is easy to see from the biopsy reports that the presence of localized foci of pathology should be included in the differential diagnosis of these facial pain patients.

Necrotic and infected pulp tissue left in root canal-treated teeth, bacteria within the root canal spaces and dentinal tubules, osteonecrotic/osteomyelitic bone with the presence of bacterial colonies, bone marrow edema, granulomas, and cysts are some of the pathological conditions that can have both a local and systemic effect. Microscopic tissue examination can detect the presence of disease that is routinely missed by typical dental exams.

Protocol for Optimal Health

Overview

While the aim of this book is to make clear the negative health consequences of root canal-treated teeth, periodontal disease, and cavitations, this chapter will attempt to give the reader an optimal program for minimizing increased oxidative stress throughout the body. Increased oxidative stress is involved in the genesis, maintenance, and progression of all diseases, and the more effectively that this oxidative stress is chronically minimized, the better health will be.

Even though it is never recommended to have the root canal procedure or to leave existing root canal-treated teeth in the mouth, it is realized that many people will opt to keep their root canal-treated teeth for any of a number of reasons. With this in mind, then, the following recommendations apply even more to those who leave root canal-treated teeth in their mouths, as all infections and toxins are strongly pro-oxidant, resulting in the worsening of all chronic degenerative diseases. Greater detail on the recommended protocol below is covered in an earlier book, *Death by Calcium*.

All increased oxidative stress results from increased toxin exposure and decreased antioxidant/ nutrient stores. Addressing only toxin exposure or only good nutrition and supplementation will always fall short of the goal. Nevertheless, addressing only one of the two issues is vastly better than addressing neither.

So, regardless of whether you remove your dental sources of infections and toxins, the following general recommendations are offered to help you in your quest for optimal health.

Primary Dental Issues

If you have reached this place in the book you are probably thinking that you never want to see another dentist ever again. The truth is that there are many fine dentists treating diseases of the oral cavity every day and providing a great service to their patients. Preventive dentistry such as sealants to help prevent occlusal decay, regular cleanings to prevent gum disease, and early intervention to restore areas of tooth decay all help to maintain a disease-free state in the mouth. Most importantly, diligent daily home care can prevent the occurrence or progression of dental disease so that periodontal issues and infected teeth are unlikely to develop. Consider following each of these suggestions.

1) Remove root canal-treated teeth (see Appendix D for protocol).

2) Have your dentist check for any other non-viable or infected teeth and decide if enough evidence supports monitoring a suspect tooth or extracting it.

3) Surgically debride cavitations (see Appendix D for protocol).

4) Address existing gum disease and practice the following oral hygiene procedures.

Oral Hygiene Measures

Tooth Brushing: Tooth brushing should be done at least twice daily, once in the morning and then again right before bed. An electric soft toothbrush is recommended. There are many good brands on the market. Some of the battery-powered rotary type brushes found in the supermarket or pharmacy work extremely well. With a rotary brush just hold the toothbrush in place and let the rotary action of the bristles do the work. It is important to brush all tooth surfaces as well as the gums. Place the toothbrush at a 45° angle towards the gums so that the toothbrush bristles gently slide under the gum and clean the periodontal sulcus. It should take about two minutes to thoroughly brush the entire mouth. Any less time and you are probably not doing a sufficient job.

Flossing: Flossing is recommended to manually debride the sides of the tooth and the interproximal gingival sulcus where tooth brushing does not reach. Flossing once daily at bedtime with thin unwaxed dental floss is a good routine. Floss between all the teeth, taking care to run the floss against the surface of both adjacent teeth. Do not pull the floss back up and out. Instead pull the floss out the side. This prevents the re-deposit of plaque and foodstuff at the contact point of the adjacent teeth. Use a clean section of floss for each area cleaned. If your flossing causes gum bleeding, you are doing it wrong, or you need to first improve the general health of your gums with the oral water irrigation routine described below.

Oral Water Irrigation: Oral water irrigation, known to many as the Waterpik®, is essential for restoring and maintaining gum health. Nothing else really does the job that good water irrigation achieves. If you have ever brushed and flossed and then immediately used a Waterpik®, you likely saw bits of food debris still coming out in spite of your being thorough in your cleaning efforts. That is because a focal and high-pressure water jet gets to places that brushing and flossing simply cannot. Set the Waterpik® on medium intensity. Direct the flow of water in between the teeth and towards the gums so that the water is squirted into the gingival sulcus (space between the tooth and gum). The water stream will flush out any food. If used daily, it will prevent the maturation of plaque on the root surface. If your gums bleed, go to a lower pressure level and work your way up. Many people will go from bleeding significantly at low pressure levels to not bleeding at all at the highest pressure levels after a few weeks. This is a clear indicator of significantly improved gum health.

The water stream will also disrupt the bacterial colonies present under the gum and prevent them from establishing mature colonies, thereby significantly lessening the chances of developing gum disease. We also recommend adding natural non-alcohol containing mouthwash to the Waterpik® water reservoir. Fill the reservoir ¾ full with warm water and fill the remaining ¼ with mouthwash. After about one week of daily use, you should see significant improvement in gingival (gum) health and appearance. When trying to reverse existing gum disease, adding a tablespoon of 3% hydrogen peroxide to the reservoir is a good idea.

Note: Waterpik® use is especially important around dental implants. The gingival tissue around dental implants does not insert into the implant post in the same way that the gingival fibers insert into the tooth root surface. As a result, any inflammation of the gingival tissue around dental implant posts allows easy access for bacteria to migrate into the jawbone. Keeping the gingival tissue around dental implants healthy and free of inflammation is essential in the long-term success of the implant.

Cosmetic Dentistry

This is a sensitive issue. Everyone wants a beautiful smile and there are amazing things that can be done with cosmetic dentistry. Tooth veneers can dramatically improve your smile with a fraction of the tooth preparation that is needed for crowns. Therefore the risk of inducing pulp damage from a veneer is relatively low. However it is our opinion that "if it ain't broke, don't fix it."

What we mean by this is that any time you touch a tooth with a dental drill, you are causing damage to the tooth. The more extensive the procedure, such as for a crown (cap) where all of the enamel and some of the dentin is removed from the tooth, the more chance the pulp tissue will die. Further, even the best crown margins (the interface between the crown and the natural tooth) can leak over time allowing bacteria to get under the crown causing decay and eventually infection of the pulp.

In short, the least amount of dentistry required in repairing decay the better. Nothing is as good as a vital natural tooth. The minute you cut into the tooth it becomes compromised. See your dentist regularly to diagnose and treat decay early, thereby keeping filling size to a minimum and preserving the maximum amount of natural tooth structure. Cleanings every six months will help to keep the periodontal tissues in tiptop shape.

Good Health Protocol

Goals of a good health protocol include:

1) Minimize new toxin exposure (dental toxicity is usually the dominant source in most people)

2) Eradicate acute and chronic infections (this would include chronically-infected tonsils, even after root canal-treated teeth have been extracted)

3) Eliminate accumulated toxins (involves any of a variety of chelators and other toxin mobilizers, such as sweating in a sauna)

4) Improve or normalize critical regulatory hormones (testosterone, estrogen, and thyroid)

5) Optimize antioxidant and nutrient levels, especially vitamin C

6) Appropriate use of prescription medicine (modern medicine can help at times when meeting the first five goals does not completely do the job)

Suggested Supplementation

Supplement	Daily Oral Dose	Special Instructions
Vitamin C as sodium ascorbate or ascorbic acid	6,000 to 15,000 mg	Depending upon bowel tolerance, in two to four divided doses throughout the day
Vitamin C in liposome-encapsulated form	1,000 to 2,000 mg	
Vitamin C in a fat-soluble form as ascorbyl palmitate	1,000 to 2,000 mg	Divided into two doses
Lysine	5,000 mg	Divided into two doses
Proline	1,000 mg	Divided into two doses
Vitamin D3	5,000 units (Starting Dose!)	Adjust by blood testing to stay as close to a 50 ng/cc blood level as possible over time
Vitamin K2 (menaquinone-4, or menatetrenone)	3 to 6 mg	
Magnesium glycinate	400 mg	Divided into two doses
Omega-3 fish oil (EPA and DHA content)	1 to 2 grams	Divided into two doses

Supplement	Daily Oral Dose	Special Instructions
Mixed tocopherols (vitamin E source)	800 IU	Divided into two doses
Beta carotene (vitamin A source)	25,000 to 50,000 IU	
Complete B vitamin complex (as from Life Extension Foundation)	1 to 2 Capsules	Divided into two doses if taking 2 capsules
Specifically AVOID any supplementation with copper, calcium, or iron; iron should only be taken for laboratory-documented iron deficiency anemia		

Beyond the scope of this book, but covered in *Death by Calcium*, are included the ways to best track diseases and their response to therapy, along with the most important laboratory testing that needs to be followed.

Remember that you need to be completely in charge of your health, and a good physician will work with you to achieve this goal.

How Insurance Companies Influence Dental Care

This book has presented a legitimate and compelling scientific case supporting the consistent toxicity found in root canal-treated teeth, as well as the pathology found in a dental entity known as the cavitation. The case has also been made in this book that the common, and decidedly not rare, cavitation should be surgically debrided, just like a pocket of infection and necrosis should be debrided anywhere else in the body. Until powerful industries like the insurance companies are willing to support the scientific truth, the dental profession will continue to attack or ignore this evidence.

The insurance industry provides stark proof of this reality. As an example, a major insurance company (Aetna) decided that the surgical treatment of the cavitation, as found in the mouths of many people, was something for which it did want to pay the treating dentist.

In addition to denying such reimbursement, Aetna also attempted to question the legitimacy of the pathology involved in the cavitation. It even recommended dental board action against any dentist treating this dental condition, a truly incredible overreach for an entity not performing the dental work. In so doing this company, as well as other insurance companies, have played a major role in causing modern dentistry to simply deny that the cavitation is both a commonly occurring and toxic dental entity.

Because of the influence that major insurance companies wield, it would seem that it is a lot easier for busy dentists to just dismiss the existence of cavitations and defer to those companies to decide the dental standard of care and the legitimacy of different aspects of dental science.

Aetna Insurance Company's Clinical Policy Bulletin Number 0642 titled "Neuralgia Inducing Cavitational Osteonecrosis (NICO) and Ultrasonograph Densitometer to Detect NICO" is representative of the immense pressure the insurance industry exerts against the extraction of root canal-treated teeth, the acknowledgment of the cavitation as a common and pathologic bone condition, and the need for the surgical debridement of the cavitation.

Excerpts from the policy bulletin will be followed with a point-by-point analysis.

Legitimacy of Cavitation Interventions

Aetna considers the surgical debridement of cavitations to be experimental and investigational, while questioning the clinical significance of NICO itself. NICO is the professional name ascribed to the subset of cavitations that cause pain. Although cavitations are very real, as discussed in Chapter 12 and shown in photos included in this book, the dental industry refuses to acknowledge the clinical significance of cavitations, and therefore it dismisses any need for treating them. Some dentists even deny their very existence. Here's what the policy bulletin states about the subject:

> Aetna considers surgery (including scraping of "infected cavities" and removal of root-canal-treated teeth) and/or any other therapies (e.g., rinsing the "cavity" with colloidal silver and administering chelation therapy and intravenous vitamin C) and bone graft replacement for the treatment of neuralgia inducing cavitational osteonecrosis (NICO)-related diagnoses to be experimental and investigational because the clinical significance of this syndrome is in question.

Counterpoint: Cavitations and NICO have been known for a very long time and this has been scientifically—as well as photographically documented—throughout this book. All of the cases that report resolution of pain after surgical debridement of cavitations further support that a cavitation is a real diagnosis. Further, most of the cavitations do NOT cause pain. So, classifying all cavitations as NICO is misleading, since by definition neuralgia means pain. Still, Aetna, the ADA, and most practicing dentists refuse to recognize that cavitations and NICO actually exist as pathologic conditions. Further, dentists and physicians who do treat NICO and cavitations can potentially be brought up on misconduct charges by state licensing boards with penalties of license revocation, while also facing accusations of insurance fraud.

Aetna is correct, however, in asserting that the administration of anything other than those medicaments routinely accepted in orthopedic surgery is not advocated. However, that is a distinct and separate issue from the surgical debridement of osteonecrotic bone.

Use of Devices to Diagnose Pain-Inducing Cavitations (NICO) or NICO-type Conditions

Since the clinical significance of NICO has been deemed "questionable," diagnosis of this condition is also "questionable," and therefore, is not sanctioned by Aetna. Here's what the policy bulletin states:

> Aetna considers the use of devices to image the jawbones to diagnose NICO or NICO-type conditions experimental and investigational because there is no adequate scientific evidence to support their clinical value.

Counterpoint: The authors of this book have never advocated the use of any device other than X-rays to diagnose cavitations. As has been shown, 3D cone beam X-ray imaging can now definitively detect cavitations where 2D X-rays might not.

Diagnosis of NICO and Claims of Cure for Systemic Diseases

Aetna and others try to discredit the significance of NICO by referencing a single study that supports its conclusion and by referencing the fact that some dentists make unsupported curative claims concerning removal of cavitations with this statement:

> The clinical significance of "neuralgia inducing cavitational osteonecrosis" (NICO), or cavitational osteopathosis, has been called into question. Dodes and Schissel (2000) reviewed the history of this syndrome. They explained that the American Academy of Biological Dentistry and other proponents of NICO claim that facial pain is caused by infected "cavities" within the jawbones. In addition, some proponents claim they can cure such conditions as arthritis, heart disease, and pain throughout the body by removing these infected cavities from the patient's jawbones. Unlike abscesses, cysts, or periapical lesions, these cavities are not apparent on X-ray films, but are only purportedly detectable with an ultrasonograph bone densitometer.

Counterpoint: Ethical dentists who treat cavitations DO NOT claim that they can cure diseases such as heart disease, arthritis, and pain throughout the body. Yes, sometimes improvements in these conditions do occur after the debridement of cavitations. The reason this book recommends the removal of infected root canal-treated teeth and the debridement of cavitations is to remove sources of infectious and toxic stress on the body. If these dental foci were factors in sustaining or worsening any systemic diseases in the patients being treated, then improvements may occur.

Contrary to the claim of Dodes and Schissel, these lesions DO appear on 3D cone beam imaging. Why they are less apparent on 2D X-ray (although many still can be seen) has been explained in the chapter on cavitations. Perhaps Dodes and Schissel had not worked with 3D cone beam imaging on cavitated areas of the jawbone when they made their assertions, since their paper was published 14 years ago.

Treatment of Chronic Pain Attributed to NICO

Aetna and others suggest that the chronic pain attributed to NICO is simply a problem with nerves and not associated with the presence of infected and necrotic tissue in tooth extraction sites. They state:

Klassner and Epstein (2011) reviewed the literature for NICO, and stated that "the etiology, pathogenesis and treatment of NICO are speculative and not well defined, and the reported bone changes may represent variations of normal changes. As a result, one can argue that the symptoms of chronic pain attributed to NICO are better explained by established concepts of neuropathic pain; thus, they should be approached medically and not managed surgically." The authors concluded: "Without a confirmed clinical diagnosis of localized bone pathosis, aggressive and invasive procedures are not warranted. Such interventions may have no effect or may even worsen the pain by increasing sensitization of the central nervous system."

Counterpoint: The proposed cause of the neuropathic pain in NICO is the toxic elements within the cavitation itself damaging the nerves. Pain is just a symptom of the underlying pathology. The cavitation is the cause of the toxicity resulting in neuropathic pain. Treating only the symptom (pain), without treating the cause (cavitation), makes no sense at all. Unless Klassner and Epstein have figured out how to make dead bone alive again, their claim that NICO should be treated medically instead of surgically is patently absurd. Further, there are an abundance of case reports showing resolution of pain after surgical debridement of NICO lesions. Contrary to their statement, there is diagnosis confirmation and documentation of bone pathology. It is unclear how Klassner and Epstein came to their conclusion. Although there is the risk of pain getting worse after surgery, this risk is minimal. All surgical procedures have risk. Perhaps most amazing is how Klassner and Epstein can make these ridiculous assertions with the existence of multiple pictures clearly documenting the necrotic breakdown that is part of the cavitation process, as demonstrated in this book. (See Chapter 12 and Appendix B.)

Extraction of Root Canal-Treated Teeth and Surgical Intervention in Treatment of NICO

Aetna and the AAE declare that both the extraction of root canal-treated teeth and the surgical intervention in the treatment of NICO are unethical and should be reported. They state:

> In a position statement, the American Association of Endodontists (AAE, 2012) has stated that the association "cannot condone surgical interventions intended to treat suspected NICO lesions... In addition, the practice of recommending the extraction of endodontically treated teeth for the prevention of NICO, or any other disease, is unethical and should be reported immediately to the appropriate state board of dentistry."

Counterpoint: This last statement says it all. The AAE refuses to recognize the diagnosis of NICO, cavitations, or the systemic disease risks of root canal-treated teeth.

It is true that some practitioners claim the ability to cure a whole host of systemic diseases by extracting root canal-treated teeth and surgically debriding cavitations. The authors strongly disagree with this practice and agree that this constitutes misconduct. However, that does not mean that removal of dead, infected root canal-treated teeth and/or surgical debridement of dead and infected bone, as in cavitation surgery, is misconduct or fraud. It just means that just like a host of other medical conditions, direct causation cannot be proven. It is simply a procedure to remove dead and infected tissue from the body, something that is considered malpractice to *AVOID* if those infections and pockets of necrosis are anywhere in the body outside of the jawbone.

By making a blanket statement denying the pathology of NICO lesions and the systemic risks of root canal-treated teeth, it would appear that Aetna disagrees with most, if not all, of the scientific research presented in this book. Furthermore, they deem any dentists who are aware of this research and appropriately extract root canal-treated teeth and debride cavitations as being unethical and deserving of having their licenses to practice revoked by their state licensing boards.

It seems that the AAE would rather protect its own interests, which is focused entirely on promoting the safety and the utilization of the root canal procedure, than the interests of the public. The AAE

refuses to do any substantive research on the systemic risks of root canal-treated teeth, as well as
cavitations, and instead it stands behind false models of safety while ignoring all of the evidence to the
contrary.

Recommended Reading and Resources

Books by Dr. Levy

Uninformed Consent: The Hidden Dangers in Dental Care,
   (with Hal A. Huggins, DDS, MS), Hampton Roads Publishing
   Company, Inc., Charlottesville, VA, 1999
Optimal Nutrition for Optimal Health,
   McGraw-Hill (Keats Publishing), New York, NY, 2001
The Roots of Disease: Connecting Dentistry and Medicine,
   (with Robert Kulacz, DDS) Xlibris Corporation, Philadelphia, PA, 2002
Curing the Incurable: Vitamin C, Infectious Diseases, and Toxins,
   MedFox Publishing, Henderson, NV, 2002
Stop America's #1 Killer, MedFox Publishing, Henderson, NV, 2006
GSH: Master Defender Against Disease, Toxins, and Aging,
   MedFox Publishing, Henderson, NV, 2008
Living in Your Right Mind, MedFox Publishing, Henderson, NV, 2010
Primal Panacea, MedFox Publishing, Henderson, NV, 2011
*Death by Calcium: Proof of the Toxic Effects of Dairy and Calcium
   Supplements,* MedFox Publishing, Henderson, NV, 2013

Website and Blog by Dr. Kulacz
   www.coletrex.com
   www.toxictooth.com (blog)

Serum Biocompatibility Testing
This is to help minimize the toxicity of dental materials and products
to be used in your dental treatments: http://www.shslab.com/

Physicians

A doctor who might be open to some or all of the treatment options discussed in this book:

 www.acamnet.org
 orthomolecular.org
 www.a4m.com
 www.icimed.com
 www.acimconnect.com
 www.grossmanwellness.com

Quality Products and Supplements

Find health products like those discussed in this book:

 www.vitaminc.com
 www.lef.org
 www.livonlabs.com
 www.altrient-europe.com
 www.swansonvitamins.com
 www.mcguff.com
 torrancecompany.com
 hightechhealth.com
 www.meritpharm.com

Further Information and for Medical Care:

 www.doctoryourself.com
 gordonresearch.com
 riordanclinic.org
 http://fluoridealert.org
 Dental infections volume 1 and 2 by Weston Price, DDS
  http://ppnf.org/product/books-1/dental-infections-
  volume-one-and-two/
 www.vitamincfoundation.org
 www.drwhitaker.com
 peakenergy.com (info and help finding a dentist)
 www.medfoxpub.com
 www.oasisofhope.com
 www.patrickholford.com
 www.naturalhealth365.com
 www.garynull.com
 naturalnews.com

These websites are for general reference only, and any information or treatments that might result from their use cannot be guaranteed to be in complete agreement with the information provided in this book. In fact, consider bringing this book to the attention of any dentist, physician, or other healthcare provider who you decide to see as a patient.

References

Introduction

1. http://www.aae.org/patients/treatments-and-procedures/root-canals/myths-about-root-canals-and-root-canal-pain.aspxls/root-canals.aspx

2. Ross, Lee; Anderson, Craig A, "Shortcomings in the attribution process: on the origins and maintenance of erroneous social assessments", in Kaheneman, Daniel; Slovic, Paul, Tversky, Amos, *Judgements under uncertainity: Heuristics and biasis, Cambridge* University Press, 1982, pp 129-152, ISBS 978-0-521-28414-1 OCLC 7579020.

Chapter One

1. http://www.aae.org/patients/treatments-and-procedures/root-canals/root-canals.aspx

Chapter Two

1. Rotstein I., Salehrabi R, "Endodontic treatment outcomes in a large patient population in the USA: an epidemiological study", *Journal of Endodontics* (2004) 12 (30): 846–50.

2. http://www.aae.org/patients/treatments-and-procedures/root-canals/myths-about-root-canals-and-root-canal-pain.aspx

3. Misra A, Spencer P, Marangos O, Wang Y, Katz JL, "Parametric study of the effect of phase anisotropy on the micromechanical behaviour of dentin–adhesive interfaces," *Royal Society Publishing*, 2005.

4. http://www.ext.colostate.edu/pubs/foodnut/kitchen-sanitize.pdf

5. Ruschel HC, Chevitarese O, "Density and diameter of dentinal tubules of first and second primary human molars—comparative scanning electron microscopy study," *J Clin Pediatr Dent.* 2002 Spring;26(3):297-304.

6. Shashidhar C, et al, "The comparison of microbial leakage in roots filled with resilon and gutta-percha: An *in vitro* study," *J Conserv Dent.* 2011 Jan-Mar; 14(1): 21–27.

7. Shantiaee Y, et al, "Comparing Microleakage in Root Canals Obturated with Nanosilver Coated Gutta-Percha to Standard Gutta-Percha by Two Different Methods," *Iran Endod J.* 2011 Autumn; 6(4): 140–145.

Chapter Three

1. Shashidhar C, et al, "The comparison of microbial leakage in roots filled with resilon and gutta-percha: An *in vitro* study," *J Conserv Dent.* 2011 Jan-Mar; 14(1): 21–27.

2. Shantiaee Y, et al, "Comparing Microleakage in Root Canals Obturated with Nanosilver Coated Gutta-Percha to Standard Gutta-Percha by Two Different Methods," *Iran Endod J.* 2011 Autumn; 6(4): 140–145.

3. Price WA, *Dental Infections Oral and Systemic, Volume I, Part I*, Price-Pottenger Nutrition Foundation, La Mesa, CA. 1923; 35-54.

4. De Moor RJ, Hommez GM, De Boever JG, Delmé KI, Martens GE, "Periapical health related to the quality of root canal treatment in a Belgian population," *Int Endod J.* 2000;33:113–20.

5. Saunders WP, Saunders EM, "Prevalence of periradicular periodontitis associated with crowned teeth in an adult Scottish subpopulation," *Br Dent J.* 1998;185:137–40.

6. Gündüz K, Avsever H, Orhan, K, Demirkaya K, "Cross-sectional evaluation of the periapical status as related to quality of root canal fillings and coronal restorations in a rural adult male population of Turkey," *BMC Oral Health*, 2011; 11:20.

7. Weiger R, Hitzler S, Hermle G, Löst C, "Periapical status, quality of root canal fillings and estimated endodontic treatment needs in an urban German population," *Endod Dent Traumatol.* 1997;13:69–74.

8. Gündüz K, Avsever H, Orhan, K, Demirkaya K, "Cross-sectional evaluation of the periapical status as related to quality of root canal fillings and coronal restorations in a rural adult male population of Turkey," *BMC Oral Health*, 2011; 11:20.

9. Lofthag-Hansen S, Huumonen S, Grondahl K, Grondahl H, "Limited cone-beam CT and intraoral radiography for the diagnosis of periapical pathology," *Oral Surgery, Oral Medicine, Oral Pathology, Oral Radiology, and Endodontics*, 2007, 103:114-119. PMID: 17178504

10. Anderson P, Yong R, Surman T et al, "Application of three-dimensional computed tomography in craniofacial clinical practice and research," *Australian Dental Journal*, 2014 Feb 24. [Epub ahead of print] PMID: 24611727

11. Adrians PA, DeBoever JA, Loesche W, "Bacterial invasion in root cementum and radicular dentin of periodontally diseased teeth in humans: A reservoir of periodontopathic bacteria," *Journal of Periodontology*, 1988 (59) 222-230.

12. http://www.aae.org/patients/treatments-and-procedures/root-canals/myths-about-root-canals-and-root-canal-pain.aspx

Chapter Four

1. Adriaens PA, De Boever JA, Loesche WJ, "Bacterial invasion in root cementum and radicular dentin of periodontally diseased teeth in humans. A reservoir of periodontopathic bacteria," *J Periodontol.* 1988 Apr;59(4):222-30. PMID: 3164373.

2. http://www.aae.org/patients/treatments-and-procedures/root-canals/myths-about-root-canals-and-root-canal-pain.aspx

3. *Cecil Textbook of Medicine 19th edition*, W B Saunders Co, Philadelphia, PA, 1991.

Chapter Five

1. http://www.aae.org/patients/treatments-and-procedures/root-canals/myths-about-root-canals-and-root-canal-pain.aspx

2. Mayo, CH, *The Dental Cosmos*, 57:899-900, 1913.

3. Shakman SH, *Medicine's Grandest Fraud, PhD Dissertation Exposing an Elaborate 1928 Fraud and Pervasive Impacts on Modern Medicine and Dentistry*, Institute of Science, 2004, instituteofscience.com.

4. Cecil, RL, and Angevine, DM, *Ann Int Med*, 12, 577, 1938.

5. Rocas I, Siqueira J, Debelian G, "Analysis of symptomatic and asymptomatic primary root canal infections in adult Norwegian patients," *Journal of Endodontics*, 2011, 37:1206-1212. PMID: 21846535

6. Siqueira J, Rocas I, "Diversity of endodontic microbiota revisited," *Journal of Dental Research*, 2009 88:969-981. PMID: 19828883

7. Siqueira J, Rocas I, "Microbiology and treatment of acute apical abscesses," *Clinical Microbiology Reviews*, 2013, 26:255-273. PMID: 23554416

8. Nobrega L, Delboni M, Martinho F et al, "Treponema diversity in root canals with endodontic failure," *European Journal of Dentistry*, 2013 7:61-68. PMID: 23408792

9. Martinho F, Chiesa W, Zaia A, "Comparison of endotoxin levels in previous studies on primary endodontic infections," *Journal of Endodontics*, 2011 37:163-167. PMID: 21238796

10. Gomes B, Endo M, Martinho F, "Comparison of endotoxin levels found in primary and secondary endodontic infections," *Journal of Endodontics*, 2012 38:1082-1086. PMID: 22794210

11. Heasman P, "An endodontic conundrum: the association between pulpal infection and periodontal disease," *British Dental Journal*, 2014 216:275-279. PMID: 24651332

12. De Moor RJ, Hommez GM, De Boever JG, Delmé KI, Martens GE, "Periapical health related to the quality of root canal treatment in a Belgian population," *Int Endod J*, 2000;33:113–20.

13. Lofthag-Hansen S, Huumonen S, Grondahl K, Grondahl H, "Limited cone-beam CT and intraoral radiography for the diagnosis of periapical pathology," *Oral Surgery, Oral Medicine, Oral Pathology, Oral Radiology, and Endodontics*, 2007 103:114-119. PMID: 17178504

14. Adrians PA, DeBoever JA, Loesche W, "Bacterial invasion in root cementum and radicular dentin of periodontally diseased teeth in humans: A reservoir of periodontopathic bacteria," *Journal of Periodontology*, 1988 (59) 222-230.

15. http://www.aae.org/patients/treatments-and-procedures/root-canals/myths-about-root-canals-and-root-canal-pain.aspx

16. Jin LJ, Chiu GK, Corbet EF, "Are periodontal diseases risk factors for certain systemic disorders—what matters to medical practitioners?" *Hong Kong Med J*, 2003 Feb;91:31-7. Review. PMID: 12547954.

17. Gurav AN, "The association of periodontitis and metabolic syndrome," *Dent Res J*, 2014 Jan;111:1-10. PMID: 24688553

18. Offenbacher S. Periodontal diseases: Pathogenesis. *Ann Periodontol*. 1996;1:821–78.

19. Humphrey L, Fu R, Buckley D et al, "Periodontal disease and coronary heart disease incidence: a systemic review and meta-analysis," *Journal of General Internal Medicine*, 2008 23:2079-2086. PMID: 18807098

20. Kshirsagar A, Craig R, Moss K et al, "Periodontal disease adversely affects the survival of patients with end-stage renal disease," *Kidney International*, 2009 75:746-751. PMID: 19165177

21. Dorn J, Genco R, Grossi S et al, "Periodontal disease and recurrent cardiovascular events in survivors of myocardial infarction MI: the Western New York Acute MI Study," *Journal of Periodontology*, 2010 81:502-511. PMID: 20367093

22. Ameet M, Avneesh H, Babita R, Pramod P, "The relationship between periodontitis and systemic diseases—hype or hope?" *Journal of Clinical and Diagnostic Research*, 2013 7:758-762. PMID: 23730671

23. Hanaoka Y, Soejima H, Yasuda O et al, "Level of serum antibody against a periodontal pathogen is associated with atherosclerosis and hypertension," *Hypertension Research*, 2013 36:829-833. PMID: 23676848

24. Kodovazenitis G, Pitsavos C, Papadimitriou L et al, "Association between periodontitis and acute myocardial infarction: a case-control study of a nondiabetic population," *Journal of Periodontal Research*, 2014 49:246-252. PMID: 23713486

25. Barilli AL, Passos AD, Marin-Neto JA, Franco LJ, "Periodontal disease in patients with ischemic coronary atherosclerosis at a University Hospital, *Arq Bras Cardiol*. 2006 Dec;87(6):695-700. PMID: 17262105.

26. Tonetti MS, "Periodontitis and risk for atherosclerosis: an update on intervention trials," *J Clin Periodontol*, 2009 Jul;36 Suppl 10:15-9. PMID: 19432627.

27. Price WA, *Dental Infections and the Degenerative Diseases Volume II, Part I*, The Price-Pottenger Nutrition Foundation, Lemon Grove, CA, pp. 56-57

28. Price WA, *Dental Infections and the Degenerative Diseases Volume II, Part I*, The Price-Pottenger Nutrition Foundation, Lemon Grove, CA, p. 83.

29. Herzberg MC, Weyer MW, "Dental plaque, platelets, and cardiovascular diseases," *Annals of Periodontology*, 1998 July; Volume 3, Number 1, pp. 151-160.

30. Renvert S, Pettersson T, Ohlsson O, Persson GR, "Bacterial profile and burden of periodontal infection in subjects with a diagnosis of acute coronary syndrome," *J Periodontol*, 2006 Jul;77(7):1110-9. PMID: 16805672.

31. Herzberg MC, Meyer MW, "Effects of oral flora on platelets: possible consequences in cardiovascular disease," *Journal of Periodontology*, 1996 October; Volume 67, Number 10, Supplement, pp. 1138-1142.

32. Haraszthy VI, Zambon JJ, Trevisan M, Zeid M, Genco RJ, "Identification of periodontal pathogens in atheromatous plaques," *Journal of Periodontology*, 2000 October; Volume 71, Number 10, pp. 1554-1560.

33. Loesche WJ, "Periodontal disease as a risk factor for heart disease," *Compendium*, 1994 August; Volume 15, Number 8, pp. 976, 978-982, 985-986.

34. Mattila KJ, "Dental infections as a risk factor for acute myocardial infarction," *European Heart Journal*, 1993 December; Volume 14, Supplement K, pp. 51-53.

35. Costa T, de Figueiredo Neta J, de Oliveira A et al, "Association between chronic apical periodontitis and coronary artery disease," *Journal of Endodontics*, 2014 40:164-167. PMID: 24461397

36. Beck JD, Pankow J, Tyroler HA, Offenbacher S, "Dental infections and atherosclerosis," *American Heart Journal*, 1999 November; Volume 138, Number 5 Pt 2, pp. S528-S533.

37. Berent R, Auer J, Schmid P, "Periodontal and coronary heart disease in patients undergoing coronary angiography," *Metabolism*, 2011 60:127-133. PMID: 20096894

38. Costa T, de Figueiredo Neta J, de Oliveira A et al, "Association between chronic apical periodontitis and coronary artery disease," *Journal of Endodontics*, 2014 40:164-167. PMID: 24461397

39. Caplan D, Chasen J, Krall E et al, "Lesions of endodontic origin and risk of coronary artery disease," *Journal of Dental Research*, 2006 85:996-1000. PMID: 17062738

40. Willershausen I, Weyer V, Peter M et al, "Association between chronic periodontal and apical inflammation and acute myocardial infarction," *Odontology*, 2013 Apr 21. PMID: 23604464

41 Pasqualini D, Bergandi L, Palumbo L et al, "Association among oral health, apical periodontitis, CD14 polymorphisms, and coronary heart disease in middle-aged adults," *Journal of Endodontics*, 2012 38:1570-1577. PMID: 23146639

42. Ott S, El Mokhtari N, Musfeldt M et al, "Detection of diverse bacterial signatures in atherosclerotic lesions of patients with coronary heart disease," *Circulation*, 2006 113:929-937. PMID: 16490835

43. Ott S, El Mokhtari N, Rehman A et al, "Fungal rDNA signatures in coronary atherosclerotic plaques," *Environmental Microbiology*, 2007 9:3035-3045. PMID: 17991032

44. Pessi T, Karhunen V, Karjalainen P et al, "Bacterial signatures in thrombus aspirates of patients with myocardial infarction," *Circulation*, 2013 127:1219-1228. PMID: 23418311

45. Zaremba M, Górska R, Suwalski P, Kowalski J. "Evaluation of the incidence of periodontitis-associated bacteria in the atherosclerotic plaque of coronary blood vessels," *J Periodontol*, 2007 Feb;78(2):322-7. PMID: 17274722.

46. Pussinen PJ, Tuomisto K, Jousilahti P, Havulinna AS, Sundvall J, Salomaa V, "Endotoxemia, immune response to periodontal pathogens, and systemic inflammation associate with incident cardiovascular disease events," *Arterioscler Thromb Vasc Biol*, 2007 Jun;27(6):1433-9. PMID: 17363692.

47. Ford PJ, Gemmell E, Chan A, Carter CL, Walker PJ, Bird PS, West MJ, Cullinan MP, Seymour GJ, "Inflammation, heat shock proteins and periodontal pathogens in atherosclerosis: an immunohistologic study," *Oral Microbiol Immunol*, 2006 Aug;21(4):206-11. PMID: 16842503.

48. Caplan D, Pankow J, Cai J et al, "The relationship between self-reported history of endodontic therapy and coronary heart disease in the Atherosclerosis Risk in Communities Study," *Journal of the American Dental Association*, 2009 140:1004-1012. PMID: 19654253

49. Frisk F, Hakeberg M, Ahlqwist, Bengtsson C, "Endodontic variables and coronary artery disease," *Acta Odontologica Scandinavica*, 2003 61:257-262. PMID: 14763775

50. Joshipura K, Pitiphat W, Hung H et al, "Pulpal inflammation and incidence of coronary heart disease," *Journal of Endodontics*, 2006 32:99-103. PMID: 16427454

51. Leong X, Ng C, Badiah B, Das S, "Association between hypertension and periodontitis: possible mechanisms," *The Scientific World Journal*, 2014 2014:768237. PMID: 24526921

52. Franek E, Napora M, Blach A, Budlewski T, Gozdowski D, Jedynasty K, Krajewski J, Gorska R, "Blood pressure and left ventricular mass in subjects with type 2 diabetes and gingivitis or chronic periodontitis," *J Clin Periodontol*, 2010 Oct; 37(10):875-80.

53. Vlachopoulos C, Dima I, Aznaouridis K, Vasiliadou C, Ioakeimidis N, Aggeli C, Toutouza M, Stefanadis C, "Acute systemic inflammation increases arterial stiffness and decreases wave reflections in healthy individuals," *Circulation*, 2005 Oct 4; 112(14):2193-200.

54. Price WA, *Dental Infections and the Degenerative Diseases Volume II, Part I*, The Price-Pottenger Nutrition Foundation, Lemon Grove, CA, pp. 111.

55. Palm F, Lahdentausta L, Sorsa T et al, "Biomarkers of periodontitis and inflammation in ischemic stroke: a case-control study," *Innate Immunity*, 2013 Sep 17. PMID: 24045341

56. Slowik J, Wnuk M, Grzech K et al, "Periodontitis affects neurological deficit in acute stroke," *Journal of the Neurological Sciences*, 2010 297:82-84. PMID: 20723913

57. Jimenez M, Krall E, Garcia R et al, "Periodontitis and incidence of cerebrovascular disease in men," *Annals of Neurology*, 2009 66:505-512. PMID: 19847898

58. Söder PO, Söder B, Nowak J, Jogestrand T, "Early carotid atherosclerosis in subjects with periodontal diseases," *Stroke*, 2005 Jun;36(6):1195-200. PMID: 15879347.

59. Iwai T, "Periodontal bacteremia and various vascular diseases," *Journal of Periodontal Research*, 2009 44:689-694. PMID: 19874452

60. Marques da Silva R, Caugant DA, Eribe ER, Aas JA, Lingaas PS, Geiran O, Tronstad L, Olsen I, "Bacterial diversity in aortic aneurysms determined by 16S ribosomal RNA gene analysis," *J Vasc Surg*, 2006 Nov;44(5):1055-60. PMID: 17098542.

61. Sandi R, Pol K, Basavaraj P et al, "Association of serum cholesterol, triglyceride, high and low density lipoprotein HDL and LDL levels in chronic periodontitis subjects with risk for cardiovascular disease CVD: a cross sectional study," *Journal of Clinical and Diagnostic Research*, 2014 8:214-216. PMID: 24596778

62. Cutler CW, Shinedling EA, Nunn M, Jotwani R, Kim BO, Nares S, Iacopino AM, "Association between periodontitis and hyperlipidemia: cause or effect?," *J Periodontol*, 1999 Dec; 70(12):1429-34.

63. Lösche W, Karapetow F, Pohl A, Pohl C, Kocher T, "Plasma lipid and blood glucose levels in patients with destructive periodontal disease," *J Clin Periodontol*, 2000 Aug; 27(8):537-41.

64. Katz J, Chaushu G, Sharabi Y, "On the association between hypercholesterolemia, cardiovascular disease and severe periodontal disease, *J Clin Periodontol*, 2001 Sep; 28(9):865-8.

65. Machado AC, Quirino MR, Nascimento LF, "Relation between chronic periodontal disease and plasmatic levels of triglycerides, total cholesterol and fractions," *Braz Oral Res*, 2005 Oct-Dec; 19(4):284-9.

66. Price WA, *Dental Infections and the Degenerative Diseases Volume II, Part I*, The Price-Pottenger Nutrition Foundation, Lemon Grove, CA, pp. 54-111.

67. Gomes-Filho I, Leitao de Oliveira T, da Cruz S et al, "The influence of periodontitis in the development of nosocomial pneumonia: a case control study," *Journal of Periodontology*, 2013 Oct 30. PMID: 24171504

68. Dev Y, Goyal O, "Recurrent lung infection due to chronic peri-odontitis," *Journal of the Indian Medical Association*, 2013 111:127,129. PMID: 24003573

69. Shiota Y, Taniguchi A, Yuzurio S et al, "Septic pulmonary embolism induced by dental infection," *Acta Medica Okayama*, 2013 67:253-258. PMID: 23970324

70. Zhou X, Han J, Liu Z et al, "Effects of periodontal treatment on lung function and exacerbation frequency in patients with chronic obstructive pulmonary disease and chronic periodontitis: a 2-year pilot randomized controlled trial," *Journal of Clinical Periodontology*, 2014 Mar 4. PMID: 24593836

71. Gomes-Filho I, Soledade-Marques K, Seixas da Cruz S et al, "Does periodontal infection have an effect on severe asthma in adults?" *Journal of Periodontology*, 2013 Nov 14. PMID: 24224961

72. Price WA, *Dental Infections and the Degenerative Diseases Volume II, Part I*, The Price-Pottenger Nutrition Foundation, Lemon Grove, CA, pp. 153.

73. Nibali L, D'Aiuto F, Griffiths G, Patel K, Suvan J, Tonetti MS, "Severe periodontitis is associated with systemic inflammation and a dysmetabolic status: a case-control study," *J Clin Periodontol*, 2007 Nov; 34(11):931-7.

74. Shimazaki Y, Saito T, Yonemoto K, Kiyohara Y, Iida M, Yamashita Y, "Relationship of metabolic syndrome to periodontal disease in Japanese women: the Hisayama Study," *J Dent Res*, 2007 Mar; 86(3):271-5.

75. Furuta M, Shimazaki Y, Takeshita T et al, "Gender differences in the association between metabolic syndrome and periodontal disease: the Hisayama Study," *Journal of Clinical Periodontology*, 2013 40:743-752. PMID: 23829196

76. D'Aiuto F, Sabbah W, Netuveli G, Donos N, Hingorani AD, Deanfield J, Tsakos G, "Association of the metabolic syndrome with severe periodontitis in a large U.S. population-based survey," *J Clin Endocrinol Metab*, 2008 Oct; 93(10):3989-94.

77. Bullon P, Jaramillo R, Santos-Garcia R et al, "Relation of periodontitis and metabolic syndrome with gestational glucose metabolism disorder," *Journal of Periodontology*, 2014 85:e1-e8. PMID: 23952077

78. Khader Y, Khassawneh B, Obeidat B, Hammad M, El-Salem K, Bawadi H, Al-akour N, "Periodontal status of patients with metabolic syndrome compared to those without metabolic syndrome," *J Periodontol*, 2008 Nov; 79(11):2048-53.

79. Morita T, Ogawa Y, Takada K, Nishinoue N, Sasaki Y, Motohashi M, Maeno M, "Association between periodontal disease and metabolic syndrome," *J Public Health Dent*, 2009 Fall; 69(4):248-53.

80. Longo P, Artese H, Rabelo M, "Serum levels of inflammatory markers in type 2 diabetes patients with chronic periodontitis," *Journal of Applied Oral Science*, 2014 22:103-108. PMID: 24676580

81. Levine R, "Obesity, diabetes and periodontitis—a triangular relationship?" *British Dental Journal*, 2013 215:35-39. PMID: 23846063

82. Price WA, *Dental Infections and the Degenerative Diseases Volume II, Part II*, The Price-Pottenger Nutrition Foundation, Lemon Grove, CA, p. 279.

83. Price WA, "Dental infections, their dangers and prevention," *Radiology*, 1928 May, p.89.

84. Price WA, *Dental Infections and the Degenerative Diseases Volume II, Part II*, The Price-Pottenger Nutrition Foundation, Lemon Grove, CA, p. 328.

85. Costa A, Yasuda C, Shibasaki W et al, "The association between periodontal disease and seizure severity in refractory epilepsy patients," *Seizure*, 2014 23:227-230. PMID: 24456623

86. Sparks Stein P, Steffen M, Smith C et al, "Serum antibodies to periodontal pathogens are a risk factor for Alzheimer's disease," *Alzheimer's & Dementia*, 2012 8:196-203. PMID: 22546352

87. Slowik J, Wnuk M, Grzech K et al, "Periodontitis affects neurological deficit in acute stroke," *Journal of the Neurological Sciences*, 2010 297:82-84. PMID: 20723913

88. Price WA, *Dental Infections and the Degenerative Diseases Volume II, Part I*, The Price-Pottenger Nutrition Foundation, Lemon Grove, CA, p. 175.

89. Ogrendik M, "Rheumatoid arthritis is an autoimmune disease caused by periodontal pathogens," *International Journal of General Medicine*, 2013 6:383-386. PMID: 23737674

90. Mikuls T, Payne J, Yu F et al, "Periodontitis and *Porphyromonas gingivalis* in patients with rheumatoid arthritis," *Arthritis and Rheumatism*, 2014 Jan 8. PMID: 24403127

91. Pendyala G, Joshi S, Chaudhari S, Gandhage D, "Links demystified: periodontitis and cancer," *Dental Research Journal*, 2013 10:704-712. PMID: 24379856

92. Michaud DS, Joshipura K, Giovannucci E, Fuchs CS, "A prospective study of periodontal disease and pancreatic cancer in US male health professionals," *J Natl Cancer Inst*, 2007 Jan 17; 99(2):171-5.

93. Stolzenberg-Solomon RZ, Dodd KW, Blaser MJ, Virtamo J, Taylor PR, Albanes D, "Tooth loss, pancreatic cancer, and *Helicobacter pylori*," *Am J Clin Nutr*, 2003 Jul; 78(1):176-81.

94. Hujoel PP, Drangsholt M, Spiekerman C, Weiss NS, "An exploration of the periodontitis-cancer association," *Ann Epidemiol*, 2003 May; 13(5):312-6.

95. Abnet CC, Qiao YL, Dawsey SM, Dong ZW, Taylor PR, Mark SD, "Tooth loss is associated with increased risk of total death and death from upper gastrointestinal cancer, heart disease, and stroke in a Chinese population-based cohort, *Int J Epidemiol*, 2005 Apr; 34(2):467-74.

96. Abnet CC, Qiao YL, Mark SD, Dong ZW, Taylor PR, Dawsey SM, "Prospective study of tooth loss and incident esophageal and gastric cancers in China," *Cancer Causes Control*, 2001 Nov; 12(9):847-54.

97. Velly AM, Franco EL, Schlecht N, Pintos J, Kowalski LP, Oliveira BV, Curado MP, "Relationship between dental factors and risk of upper aerodigestive tract cancer," *Oral Oncol*, 1998 Jul; 34(4):284-91.

98. Rosenquist K, Wennerberg J, Schildt EB, Bladström A, Göran Hansson B, Andersson G, "Oral status, oral infections and some lifestyle factors as risk factors for oral and oropharyngeal squamous cell carcinoma. A population-based case-control study in southern Sweden," *Acta Otolaryngol*, 2005 Dec; 125(12):1327-36.

99. Wen B, Tsai C, Lin C et al, "Cancer risk among gingivitis and periodontitis patients: a nationwide cohort study," *QJM*, 2014 107:283-290. PMID: 24336850

100. Kothiwale S, Desai B, Kothiwale V et al, "Periodontal disease as a potential risk factor for low birth weight and reduced maternal haemoglobin levels," *Oral Health & Preventive Dentistry*, 2014 12:83-90. PMID: 24619787

101. Fabbri C, Fuller R, Bonfa E et al, "Periodontitis treatment improves systemic lupus erythematosus response to immunosuppressive therapy," *Clinical Rheumatology*, 2014 33:505-509. PMID: 24415114

102. Anand P, Sagar D, Ashok S, Kamath K, "Association of aggressive periodontitis with reduced erythrocyte counts and reduced hemoglobin levels," *Journal of Periodontal Research*, 2013 Dec 11. PMID: 24329044

103. Barak S, Oettinger-Barak O, Machtei EE, Sprecher H, Ohel G, "Evidence of periopathogenic microorganisms in placentas of women with preeclampsia," *J Periodontol*, 2007 Apr;78(4):670-6. PMID: 17397314.

104. Alchalabi H, Al Habashneh R, Jabali O, Khader Y, "Association between periodontal disease and adverse pregnancy outcomes in a cohort of pregnant women in Jordan," *Clinical and Experimental Obstetrics & Gynecology*, 2013 40:399-402. PMID: 24283174

105. Vavricka S, Manser C, Hediger S et al, "Periodontitis and gingivitis in inflammatory bowel disease: a case-control study," *Inflammatory Bowel Diseases*, 2013 19:2768-2777. PMID: 24216685

106. Pressman G, Qasim A, Verma N et al, "Periodontal disease is an independent predictor of intracardiac calcification," *BioMed Research International*, 2013:854340. PMID: 24106721

107. Herrera B, Bastos A, Coimbra L et al, "Peripheral blood mononuclear phago-cytes from patients with chronic periodontitis are primed for osteoclast for-mation," *Journal of Periodontology,* 2013 Sep 24. PMID: 24059638

108. Wu C, Yang T, Lin H et al, "Sudden sensorineural hearing loss associated with chronic periodontitis: a population-based study," *Otology & Neurotology,* 2013 34:1380-1384. PMID: 24026022

109. Chakraborty D, Tewari D, Sharma D, Narula D, "Effect of non-surgical peri-odontal therapy on serum ferritin levels: an interventional study," *Journal of Periodontology,* 2013 Jul 4. PMID: 23826646

110. Wendling D, Prati C, "Spondyloarthritis and smoking: towards a new insight into the disease," *Expert Review of Clinical Immunology,* 2013 9:511-516. PMID: 23730882

111. Antal M, Braunitzer, Mattheos N et al, "Smoking as a permissive factor of periodontal disease in psoriasis," *PLoS One,* 2014 9:e92333. PMID: 24651659

112. Gokhale N, Acharya A, Patil V et al, "A short-term evaluation of the rela-tionship between plasma ascorbic acid levels and periodontal disease in sys-temically healthy and type 2 diabetes mellitus subjects," *Journal of Dietary Supplements,* 2013 10:93-104. PMID: 23725523

113. Bastos Jdo A, Andrade L, Ferreira A et al, "Serum levels of vitamin D and chronic periodontitis in patients with chronic kidney disease," *Jornal Brasile-iro de Nefrologia,* 2013; 35:20-26. PMID: 23598748

Chapter Six

1. http://www.aae.org/patients/treatments-and-procedures/root-canals/myths-about-root-canals-and-root-canal-pain.aspx

2. Authors Not Listed, "Root Canal Therapy Safe and Effective," Endodontics: Colleagues for Excellence, (1994) Fall/Winter, p 1.

3. Authors Not Listed, "When infection does spread from an infected root ca-nal," Endodontics: Colleagues for Excellence, (1994) Fall/Winter, p 3.

4. http://www.tupeloendo.com/pdfs/AAE-Guidlines/AAE-Position-Statme-ment-Paraformaldehyde-Filling-Materials.pdf

5. Tezal M, Scannapieco FA, Wactawski-Wende J, et al, "Dental Caries and Head and Neck Cancers," *JAMA Otolaryngol Head Neck Surg.* 2013;139(10):1054-1060.

Chapter Ten

1. Mavroudis C, Mavroudis CD, Jacobs J et al, "Procedure-based complications to guide informed consent: analysis of Society of Thoracic Surgeons-Congen-ital Heart Surgery Database," *The Annals of Thoracic Surgery,* 2014 Mar 27. [Epub ahead of print] PMID: 24680033.

Chapter Twelve

1. Levy T, Huggins H, "Routine dental extractions routinely produce cavita-tions," *Journal of Advancement in Medicine,* 1996, 9:235-249.

Robert Kulacz, DDS

Dr. Kulacz received his dental degree from New York University College of Dentisty, and he received post-graduate training in implant surgery and implant restoration sponsored by Brookdale Hospital in Brooklyn N.Y.

He abandoned much of his traditional dental practice after learning of the risks of some of the dental procedures he was performing. Subsequently, he only performed oral surgery. He has not actively practiced dentistry since 2006.

His first book, *The Roots of Disease*, with co-author Dr. Tom Levy was published in 2002. It introduced many of the concepts that *The Toxic Tooth* now greatly expands upon. It was Dr. Levy who suggested that *The Roots of Disease* be revised and updated. Reluctant at first, Dr. Kulacz finally agreed. However, soon after starting the revision, Drs. Kulacz and Levy quickly realized that the abundant new and compelling research published since 2002 warranted a complete new book: *The Toxic Tooth*.

Email: rkulacz@yahoo.com

Thomas E. Levy, MD, JD

Dr. Levy is a board-certified cardiologist and a bar-certified attorney. *The Toxic Tooth* marks his tenth health-related book. Since discontinuing the practice of traditional cardiology 20 years ago, he has focused on the importance of minimizing toxins in the body, especially those originating in the mouth, while optimizing the antioxidant capacity in the body, most prominently that of vitamin C. He lectures around the world now on a regular basis on these topics. Currently, he is involved in ongoing research efforts to validate the importance of increased oxidative stress in the genesis and worsening of all chronic degenerative diseases, along with continuing efforts to develop disease treatment protocols based on these concepts.

PeakEnergy.com
Email: televymd@yahoo.com